Contents

Editors v
Contributors...v

1. Communicating with Cancer Patients and their Families
   *Jonelle M. Farrow, PhD, D. Kaye Cash, MD, and Gretchen Sim-
   mons, MSW* 1
2. The Caring Process and the Cancer Patient
   Joan Paternoster, RN, MS 18
3. Factors that Contribute to Control and Hopefulness
   Barbara R. Breitbart, PhD..26
4. Symptom Control, Ethics, and Communication Patterns: Crucial Topics in
   Cancer Education
   Samuel C. Klagsbrun, MD 33
5. Factors Contributing to Poorly Relieved Pain in the Cancer Patient
   Nessa Coyle, RN, MS 39
6. Psychosocial Interventions with Cancer Patients and Their Families
   Francine Cournos, MD 45
7. Clinical Cancer Education in the Pediatric Setting
   Anneliese Sitarz, MD..49
8. The Cancer Educator as Role Model: A Means of Initiating Attitude Change
   Salvatore J. Bertolone, MD and Pamela Scott, RN, BSN 56
9. Cancer: A Situational Problem: A Curriculum for Health Professionals to
   Teach Children whose Parents have Cancer
   Irene Sullivan, EdD, CSW..60
10. Using Group Process and Therapeutic Metaphor in the Psychological Care
    of Pediatric Cancer Patients and Their Siblings
    Amita Jensen, PhD 77
11. Cancer: Curriculum for Well Siblings of Pediatric Cancer Patients
    Irene Sullivan, EdD, CSW..90
12. Cancer and the Family: Experiences of Children and Adolescents
    Edythe S. Ellison, RN, PhD 115
13. Breast Cancer: Living with Uncertainty
    Susan B. Westlake, RN, MS and Florence E. Selder, RN, PhD 125
14. Social Context of Breast Cancer Within the Family
    Alice L. Cullinan, PhD..134
15. Existential Group Therapy with Mastectomy Patients
    Alice L. Cullinan, PhD..150

iii

16. Cancer Communication: Education on a Head and Neck Service
    Andrew Blitzer, MD 162
17. Caring for the Patient with Head and Neck Cancer
    Mary Jo Dropkin, RN, MSN 166
18. The Role of the Head and Neck Tumor Board in Clinical Cancer Education
    Peter A. Shapiro, MD 176
19. Colon Cancer: A Prototype for Consideration of Psychosocial Aspects of Care
    Frederick Herter, MD 182
20. The Cancer Patient with Alzheimer's Disease
    Mary Ann Zubler, MD 187
21. Impact of Group Counseling on the Terminally Ill
    Calvin E. Selfridge, BA, MA 192
22. Adapting Time-Limited Therapy to the Care of Persons with Cancer
    Marilyn M. Rawnsley, DNSc 200
23. When Your Dying Becomes My Dying: Aspects of A Caregivers Grief
    Mary Dee McEvoy, RN, PhD 206
24. A Comparison of the Terminally Ill Cancer Patient's Perception of Needs vs. the Perceptions of the Family and the Nurse
    Matthew Bellanich, MS, RN 211
25. Humor as a Teaching Strategy for Caregivers
    Christine A. Rovinski, RN, MSN 218
26. The Search for an Institutional Approach to Thanatology in a Cancer Center
    Y. Silverberg, PhD, F.S. Adams, D.R. Copeland, W.L. Dorris, H. Goepfert, J.K. Levi, J.F. Stelling, K.R. Stevens and L.A. Villejos 222

Index 233

Communicating WITH Cancer Patients AND Their Families

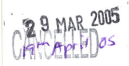
Don Gresswell Ltd., London, N21   Cat. No. 1207   DG 02242/71

This book is dedicated to the living memory of Robert Quinn.

Acknowledgment

The editors wish to acknowledge the support and encouragement of the American Institute of Life-threatening Illness and Loss, a division of the Foundation of Thanatology in the preparation of this volume. All royalties from the sale of this book are assigned to the Foundation of Thanatology, a tax exempt, not for profit, public scientific and educational foundation.

Thanatology, a new subspecialty of medicine, is involved in scientific and humanistic inquiries and the application of the knowledge derived therefrom to the subjects of the psychological aspects of dying; reactions to loss, death, and grief; and recovery from bereavement.

The Foundation of Thanatology is dedicated to advancing the cause of enlightened health care for the terminally ill patient and his family. The Foundation's orientation is a positive one based on the philosophy of fostering a more mature acceptance and understanding of death and the problems of grief and the more effective and humane management and treatment of the dying patient and his bereaved family members.

The publication of this book was supported in part by a grant from the Lucius N. Littauer Foundation.

The Charles Press
Post Office Box 15715
Philadelphia, PA 19103

Communicating with cancer patients and their families / editors,
    Andrew Blitzer . . . [et al.].
        p.   cm.
    Includes bibliographical references.
    ISBN 0-914783-33-5 : $19.95
    1. Cancer—Psychological aspects.   2. Patient education.
3. Medical personnel and patient.   I. Blitzer, Andrew.
    [DNLM: 1. Communication.   2. Family.   3. Neoplasms—psychology.
4. Patient Education.   QZ 200 C7345]
RC262.C544 1990
616.99′4′0014—dc20
DNLM/DLC   90-1554
for Library of Congress   CIP

Editors

Andrew Blitzer, MD, Professor of Clinical Otolaryngology, College of Physicians and Surgeons, Columbia University, New York.

Dr. Austin H. Kutscher, President, The Foundation of Thanatology; Professor of Dentistry (in Psychiatry), Department of Psychiatry, College of Physicians and Surgeons, Columbia University, New York.

Samuel C. Klagsbrun, MD, Associate Clinical Professor of Psychiatry, College of Physicians and Surgeons, Columbia University, New York; Director, Four Winds Hospital, Katonah, New York.

Robert DeBellis, MD, Assistant Professor of Clinical Medicine (Oncology), College of Physicians and Surgeons, Columbia University, New York.

Florence E. Selder, RN, PhD, Associate Professor and Urban Research Center Scientist, University of Wisconsin, Milwaukee, Wisconsin.

Irene B. Seeland, MD, Assistant Clinical Professor of Psychiatry, New York University Medical Center; Attending Psychiatrist, Goldwater Memorial Hospital, New York.

Mary-Ellen Siegel, MSW, ACSW, Senior Teaching Associate, Department of Community Medicine (Social Work), Mount Sinai School of Medicine, City University of New York, New York.

Contributors

Matthew Bellanich, MS, RN, Quincy, MA.

Salvatore J. Bertolone, MD, Associate Professor; Director, Pediatric Hematology/Oncology, University of Louisville, Louisville, KY.

Barbara R. Breitbart, PhD, Research Institute of Psychophysiology, NY.

D. Kay Cash, MD, Assistant Professor of Hematology/Oncology, John L. McClellan Medical Center, Little Rock, AK.

Francine Cournos, MD, Assistant Clinical Professor of Psychiatry, College of Physicians and Surgeons, Columbia University, NY.

Nessa Coyle, RN, MS, Director, Supportive Care Program, Department of Neurology, Pain Service, Memorial Sloan-Kettering Cancer Center; Instructor in Clinical Nursing, School of Nursing, Columbia University, NY.

Alice L. Cullinan, PhD, Middletown Psychiatric Center, Middletown, NY.

Mary Jo Dropkin, RN, MSN, Nurse Clinician, Head and Neck Services, Memorial Sloan-Kettering Cancer Center, NY.

Edythe S. Ellison, RN, PhD, Associate Professor and Associate Dean of Academic Affairs, College of Nursing, Department of Psychiatry, University of Illinois, Chicago.

Jonelle M. Farrow, PhD, Clinical Psychologist (Intermediate Medicine), John L. McClellan Memorial Veterans Hospital, Little Rock, AK; Adjunct Associate Professor, Family and Community Medicine, University of Arkansas for Medical Sciences.

Frederic P. Herter, MD, Auchincloss Professor Emeritus of Surgery, College of Physicians and Surgeons, Columbia University, New York; President, American University of Beirut, Beirut, Lebanon.

Amita Jensen, PhD, Psychosocial Oncology Consultant, Valley Childrens Hospital, Fresno, CA.

Mary Dee McEvoy, RN, PhD, Robert Wood Johnson Clinical Nurse Scholar, University of Pennsylvania School of Nursing, Philadelphia, PA.

Joan Paternoster, RN, MS, Pace University, Lienhard School of Nursing, Pleasantville, NY.

Marilyn M. Rawnsley, DNSc, Visiting Professor, Department of Nursing Education, Teachers College, Columbia University, New York, NY.

Christine A. Rovinski, RN, MSN, Staff Development Coordinator, Savannas Hospital, Port St. Lucie, FL.

Pamela Scott, RN, BSN, Clinical Trial Specialist, Department of Pediatric Hematology/Oncology, Kosair Children's Hospital, Louisville, KY.

Calvin Selfridge, BA, MA, HIV Counselor and Grief and Bereavement Counselor, Peter Kruger Clinic for Immunological Disorders, Beth Israel Medical Center, NY.

Peter A. Shapiro, MD, Liaison Psychiatrist to Head and Neck Service, Presbyterian Hospital; Assistant Clinical Professor of Psychiatry, Department of Psychiatry, College of Physicians and Surgeons, NY.

Yall Silverberg, PhD, Assistant Research Professor in Education Research, University of Texas System Cancer Center, M.D. Anderson Hospital and Tumor Institute, Houston, TX.

Gretchen C. Simmons, MSW, John L. McClellan Memorial Veterans Hospital, Little Rock, AK.

Anneliese L. Sitarz, MD, Professor of Clinical Pediatrics, College of Physicians, and Surgeons, Columbia University, NY.

Irene Sullivan, EdD, CSW, Instructor, Guidance and Counseling, Long Island University-Westchester Division; Private Practice, Irvington, NY.

Susan B. Westlake, RN, MS, Doctoral Candidate, University of Wisconsin-Milwaukee, Milwaukee, WI.

Mary Anne Zubler, MD, Chief of Oncology, Veterans Administration Medical Center, Houston, TX.

1

Communicating with Cancer Patients and Their Families

Jonelle M. Farrow, PhD
D. Kaye Cash, MD
Gretchen Simmons, MSW

Although we live in a sophisticated society where medical and technological advances take place almost daily, the word "cancer" (much less its actual diagnosis) still generates untold fears and anxieties. In the newly diagnosed cancer patient, the sense of loss of self-control or self-determination and the realization of his or her mortality are major factors upon which this fear of cancer is based. As Hersh (1985) so succinctly stated:

> "It (cancer) presents one's own body destroying one's self. Appearing to come from nowhere, it strikes without warning . . . Cancer represents the abnormal condition of physical self that symbolizes both our tenuous hold on life and the fragile reality of our own control" (p.55).

The diagnosis of cancer not only has a profound effect upon the patient but can also alter social interactions with family members and important others. In order to treat not only the patient's disease but the total human being, the entire health care team must be aware of how the diagnosis of cancer affects the patient's sense of self. This is where close patient communication and education play a vital role.

It is well established that education benefits cancer patients by decreasing their anxiety level (Hersh 1985). Various studies have provided insight into what specific cancer-related topics should be presented to patients and what teaching tools work best for different kinds of patients (Johnson 1982; Herzoff

1

1979; Cassileth et al. 1980, 1982; Lauer et al. 1982). The opening of our 40-bed oncology unit represented a prime opportunity for incorporating knowledge gleaned from research at various cancer institutes into a single setting. The commitment on this oncology ward is both to extend the life span and to enhance quality of life as much as feasible. A three-phase approach was outlined to address, in a holistic fashion, the needs of our cancer patients and their significant others. These three phases include:

1. *The Initial Contact:* Presenting the diagnosis to the patient and significant others;
2. *The Process of Patient Education:* Assisting the patient to live with cancer;
3. *The Terminal Phase:* Working with the dying patient. An attempt was made to achieve a well-organized educational/support system that could continue to function even in the face of frequent staff turnover— a common problem on many cancer wards. Care was taken to specifically address topics, selected on the basis of experience and research, that would benefit the patient's quality of life.

THE INITIAL CONTACT: PRESENTING THE DIAGNOSIS TO THE PATIENT AND SIGNIFICANT OTHERS

In this first phase, the physician plays the leading role. The skill with which physicians communicate information to patients and families is the most powerful tool at their disposal in helping people cope with illness. It is the physician who will begin the process of education by explaining to the patient: what the diagnosis is; what diagnostic tests are planned to define the extent of disease; recommendations for treatment; and for some patients, prognosis.

It is important that the physician who ultimately determines the treatment and care of the patient also be the one who delivers this initial information. This allows for the development of physician–patient rapport, minimizes the amount of misinformation the patient may receive, and leaves the patient with a sense that, while he is still having to come to terms with his physical condition, there is a real person who comprehends the situation and is beginning appropriate treatment. This information, therefore, not only informs but, as Cassel (1985) conceptualized, serves as a therapeutic tool in that it: (1) reduces the patient's uncertainty as to what he can expect; (2) strengthens the relationship between the physician and patient; (3) and, most importantly, may alter the patient's perception of his illness from total hopelessness to one of hope.

Not uncommonly, the patient requires a period of time to begin making adjustments and assimilating the information he has been given regarding his disease. It may only be at subsequent meetings that the patient will reveal major concerns and fears. It may, therefore, take more than one meeting with the patient for the "initial contact" phase to take place.

Another step in the initial phase is contact with the clinical psychologist, who provides assessments of all patients admitted to the ward. The aim of this initial contact is to evaluate the patient's emotional functioning, mental status, support system, and personality factors that might affect the patient's treatment program and his or her efforts to cope with cancer. One important aspect of this initial screening is to identify patients in need of immediate attention to alleviate psychological distress. For example, assessment of mood in our veteran population, especially the rural veteran, is not a quick and simple task. Patients frequently attribute symptoms such as insomnia, anorexia, sexual dysfunctioning, increased irritability, constant rumination, decreased interest, and lack of initiative to the cancer and fail to recognize that they may be experiencing a major depression. At this point, the psychologist is of invaluable aid in educating the patient as to what he is experiencing and its etiology, and helping the patient to understand that these symptoms can be addressed and improved.

Research (Schipper et al. 1984; Spitzer et al. 1981) has included ratings of "mood" as a vital feature of quality of life measures. Based on our experiences, these measures would be of suspect validity without considerable education for the patient and significant others.

Those patients who do not need to engage in psychotherapy at the initial stage of their disease learn during the interpretation of assessment results that such services are available to meet future needs. Indeed, many patients subsequently request opportunities for psychotherapy (individual or group) even though they were not self-referred for the initial assessment. Finally, the feedback session allows the psychologist to establish meaningful rapport by sharing with patients their own emotional strengths and weaknesses, which can affect efforts to cope with cancer.

Another service provided by the psychologist is neuropsychological assessment to aid in competency decisions. For example: Is the patient able to manage funds? Can he comprehend the treatment plan the physician is explaining to him? Will he be able to follow a medication regimen once discharged? On occasion, evaluation for altered mental status has allowed us to determine whether the patient is simply depressed, or whether we need to look further for brain metastases.

At times, consultation requests are made for evaluation of sexual dysfunctioning. Sexuality is of course an integral aspect of one's self-concept and represents an important part of one's life that can be disrupted by cancer and its treatment (Andersen 1985). Indeed, the American Cancer Society recently designated sexual dysfunctioning as an endpoint in psychosocial research in oncology. Sex therapy is initiated when indicated. The terminal cancer patient and his or her spouse should be the first-priority couple to be assisted in working through sexual issues and dysfunctions and evolving mutually satisfying avenues for meeting intimacy needs.

The clinical social worker, an integral member of the treatment team, contributes the philosophy of social work in regard to patient rights, knowledge of the social needs of the patients, and an evaluation of the resources for social services available in the community. The opportunities to practice several facets of social work intervention are challenging and rewarding. "Caring for the total person"—the holistic approach—is applicable as the patient and his family members indicate their needs for physical, social, psychological, and spiritual support.

The clinical social worker participates in ward rounds both with the physician and independently, to recognize and evaluate the social factors affecting each patient and, therefore, to determine the need for social worker intervention. Daily ward rounds provide a working knowledge of the patient's diagnosis, prognosis, and plans for treatment; early identification of social problems; and an opportunity to work with the patient and family to alleviate situations before they develop into crises.

Patients are encouraged to bring "other than social problems" to the social worker's attention. Frequently, patients will discuss problems related to their misunderstanding of ward routine or confusion over the purpose of medical treatments. An attempt is made to meet these concerns as simply and straightforwardly as possible with efforts to strengthen the patient's trust in the treatment plan. Concerns of the patient that can best be discussed by other professional staff are brought to the attention of those staff members.

Patient/staff liaison is a common role of the clinical social worker. Some patients express fear of their expertise relating to other staff. As one patient said, "I'm not very well educated and I don't understand some of the language used by my doctor when describing my cancer and treatment. I'm afraid to ask." It was necessary to praise this patient for his courage to say "I don't understand," and his efforts to seek an understanding. It is helpful to rehearse with such patients ways to question the physician or to ask for clarification, and most important, to encourage them to "just be yourself. You are important and so are your questions." Patients should also be encouraged to make notes to cover these concerns. This particular patient expressed added confidence that he could communicate his needs to the physician, thus relieving himself of unanswered questions and unnecessary worry.

In summary, during the initial phase patients and their families begin to become acquainted with the professional staff and the services available to assist them in coping with cancer. Data gathered by all members of the multidisciplinary team during this initial phase provide the basis for formulation of a treatment plan.

THE PROCESS OF PATIENT EDUCATION: ASSISTING THE PATIENT TO LIVE WITH CANCER

The specific goal of this second phase is to give patients factual knowledge that will help them understand what is happening to them Table-1 lists the oncology patient education series used to disseminate factual information to the patient. It is essential that patients be helped as much as possible to understand the disease process and its potential impact on them and their families. It is only through this knowledge that patients will be able to maintain a sense of control over the events taking place in their lives.

TABLE-1.
Oncology Patient Education Series.

Topic	Presenter
1. Cancer: The Disease and Treatment	Oncologist
2. Cancer Myths	Nurse
3. Radiation Therapy	Radiation Oncologist
4. Chemotherapy	Nurse Practitioner
5. Anatomy and Physiology	Nurse Practitioner
6. Helping Yourself at Home	Nurse
7. Religion	Chaplain
8. Coping with Cancer: Stress Management Sex in Health and Illness	Clinical Psychologist
9. Communication	Social Worker
10. Nutrition	Dietitian
11. Nuclear Medicine: CT Scans, X-ray	Radiologist

All members of the multidisciplinary team participate in the formal education series. In addition, the individual and group therapy sessions conducted by psychology and social work staff include educational goals as viable contributions to the therapeutic process. For example, information about the stages of grief that individuals frequently experience as they encounter losses will facilitate understanding and tolerance of the associated strong emotions in oneself and family members. At times, family members cannot or will not attend these sessions, so attempts are made to educate them through the patient. The goals of education and therapy include improved acceptance of one's physical status, emotional comfort, and enhanced quality of life. When these goals are achieved, our patients and families are able to confront death with dignity and with as little "unfinished business" as possible. As stated by Kubler-Ross (1978), they continue to "live until they say good-bye."

Individual psychotherapy is tailored to meet the individual's needs. Consequently, approaches may include dynamically oriented therapy, cognitive-behavioral therapy, hypnotherapy, crisis intervention, brief supportive therapy, grief therapy, life review therapy, or a combination of these. *Cancer, death, and dying are family systems issues, so whenever possible, all members of the immediate family are engaged in our attempts to facilitate coping with cancer; however, individual therapy may be necessary before couple or family therapy can proceed.* For example, one patient needed to deal with his feelings about dying and practice saying "I'm dying" before he was able to communicate these feelings to his wife. Consequently, after he did so, he and his wife were able to do couples therapy very rapidly and effectively. They reviewed their life together and she was able at last to say, "I can let you go now," shortly before he died.

Hypnotherapy is specifically employed to increase feelings of control and decrease feelings of helplessness, thereby improving self-esteem. Particular goals may be to control pain or side effects of treatment, help alleviate the discomfort of unpleasant procedures like bone marrow aspirates, decrease anxiety, or enhance stress management skills.

The Oncology Support Group, led by the clinical psychologist, originally was designed as a support group for our patients, but at times it is a multifamily group as well. The group process allows participants to share and model coping skills, evolve problem-solving approaches, receive emotional support from others, and provide support to others; this enables patients to help themselves and to receive satisfaction from helping others. Our group process provides patients with a community of support in addition to creating opportunities to work through feelings and fears associated with serious physical illness and facilitating the acquisition of positive coping strategies as they face the adaptive tasks encountered in dealing with their disease process. Newly diagnosed patients and their families learn from experienced patients. This adds to the support provided by our staff.

For the psychologist working with a terminal cancer patient, a unique aspect of therapy is the extent to which the psychologist must participate intimately in the patient's plight. One patient with widespread ovarian cancer and visible tumors needed for the tumors to be seen and touched. Another patient, physically disfigured by widespread melanoma, wanted his psychologist to inspect the tumors on his chest and shoulders in order to comprehend how horrible he felt about himself. One patient who was quite debilitated from his lung cancer, with bone, liver, and brain metastases, wanted to attend the weekly group therapy session, even though he was unable to hold his urine for longer than 10–15 minutes. The group process was not the least bit interrupted when he covered himself with his towel and used his urinal at frequent intervals. A patient and his wife had to share the deterioration in his condition by revealing where his cancer had literally eaten through his abdomen. It cannot be overemphasized that psychotherapy with seriously ill patients demands appreciation of their medical concerns.

Alterations in the body image (ostomies, mastectomy, hair loss secondary to chemotherapy, weight loss) and role changes can erode self-esteem. It is often necessary to remind patients that who they are has not changed. Their unique characteristics, the way they care for others, their sense of humor, and their intellect remain unchanged. But an altered body image can be devastating to one's self-esteem. One patient experienced a major depression two years after his testicles were removed during surgery for prostate cancer. His wife had never seen him nude since the surgery. He was unable to let his adult son know that his testicles had been removed. Later, in finishing his "unfinished" business, he felt safe enough to disclose feelings about his surgery to his wife and son and was proud to have told his son, for the first time ever, that he loved him.

Patience, acceptance, and sensitivity are vital components of the therapeutic process. Before psychotherapy can be initiated, it is often necessary to "normalize" the person's emotional reactions by educating them about the effect of stress on bodily functioning, the role of neurotransmitters, and the biochemical basis for depression. Goldberg (1981) has emphasized that even when there are medical conditions contributing to the psychological distress, patients need to have their emotional and personal concerns dealt with as well as their medical needs. Our patients are often told that we would have been concerned had they *not* felt the impact of this catastrophic disease. Acknowledging emotional pain, providing opportunities to express and work through feelings can facilitate the healing of emotional wounds, "normalize" reactions, and reduce the enormous burdens inherent in a terminal cancer diagnosis. In the process, the myth that depression or anxiety results from some personal weakness is destroyed.

Psychopharmacological intervention may be required before some patients can settle down to the business of psychotherapy. Our experience has not been that medications abort or delay the grief work; rather, medications, when needed, enable the person to proceed with grief work. One who is not sleeping or eating is in poor condition to tackle a life-threatening illness. It has been estimated that 20–75 percent of cancer patients have clinically significant depression (Plumb and Holland 1977; Derogatis et al. 1983; Craig and Abeloff 1974). Nevertheless, one investigator (Derogatis et al. 1979) reported that tricyclics represented only 1 percent of the psychotropics administered to cancer patients, with diazepam (Valium) being frequently prescribed. Use of Valium for depressed patients is likely to exacerbate the level of depression and increase the potential for drug toxicity, especially in elderly patients. Our psychiatry service is exceedingly helpful in assisting with psychopharmacological management of depression.

Worden and Weisman (1980) reported that approximately 33.3 percent of adult cancer patients at risk emotionally will reject intervention. Our experience has been very different, with 1 percent or less of the needy patients rejecting assistance. We feel that this marked difference in rejection rate is influenced by the nature of our program, which includes psychological services as an integral component of the everyday ward routine. In addition, because many professionals do not recognize that therapeutic encounters can be useful in treating the depression, anxiety, and adjustment problems associated with cancer, such services are either not available or, unfortunately, not offered to patients and their families. Given the evidence suggesting strongly that both quality and length of survival for cancer patients are related to psychological factors (Weisman and Worden 1975) and that psychotherapy benefits the cancer patient, (Gordon et al. 1980) careful consideration should be given to in-depth development of a psychological support system on all cancer units. Psychosocial needs of cancer patients could then be addressed.

In order to maintain staff members' ability to provide the necessary support and education for patients and to lighten the emotional burden, staff support and in-service training are important components of our program. For example, the extra stress added to the nurse's position in an oncology ward has been documented (Stewart et al. 1982).

Families experience more trauma and stress when the diagnosis is cancer than is typically realized by the cancer patients or the family members themselves. Alleviating family stress can only serve to lighten the patient's concerns. As Weisman (1976) stated, family members must be allowed to exercise such coping skills as seeking information; talking with others; and initiating positive, constructive action if they are to begin living with the diagnosis of cancer. Toward that end, a Caregiver's Support Group was organized by the social worker. This group, structured around a crisis intervention model, facilitates maximal sharing of feelings for all family members, including children, who have direct responsibility for nurturing and caring for the cancer patient. One of the more valuable sessions was attended by a patient's wife and two grandchildren, ages 11 and 15. Both children were allowed to work through feelings relative to their grandfather's impending death. They previously had not shared their feelings with their grandmother, who often stated, "I'm having to not let my grandchildren know my true feelings.'' Tears and grief were shared, and family bonds were strengthened.

Through the support group, coping behaviors are mobilized to handle the stress—increased feelings of frustration, guilt, and shock; knowledge of impending major object loss; the continuous presence of pain and suffering; futility and hopelessness—and family networking is established so the family can develop its own support system. Families are acquainted with information that strengthens their roles as caregivers and lessens the stress of living with cancer. Education decreases the frequency with which patients and family members experience anxiety, depression, and feelings of life disruption (Welch-McCaffrey 1983; Weisman 1972). Therapeutic group discussion is determined by the specific needs and crises of group members. The group provides a safe environment for the expression of powerful emotions such as anger, sadness, fear, helplessness, loneliness, and loss of control. Members often share common feelings, thus reinforcing expression of feelings. The most commonly shared emotion tends to be anger: "Why us?" Anger and shock seem to interchange. One participant said, "It just isn't fair. Just as we're about to start enjoying life we have to cope with a life-threatening illness." When someone expresses anger, shock, or dismay, others listen with the heart. Emotional relief follows the ventilation of feelings. In some cases, a participant will express spiritual beliefs related to pain and suffering and the divine power of faith. Interjection of a religious mood often moves the group toward an attitude of greater acceptance.

Family members share sentiments like, "Cancer is an unwelcome member of our family. That unwelcome family member is constantly present and is often unsightly. Sometimes it appears that it's in a state of remission but usually not for long. It's part of our daily verbal and nonverbal conversations." Families are forced to adjust to this new, constant, and unwanted family member. Feelings of aggression resulting from the amount of management and care required by the unwanted and unwelcomed family member, often surface. The role of each member may be altered by immediate changes that affect socialization, employment, and sexuality. One family member emphasized that she "could no longer socialize with friends, eating out was next to impossible, no more dancing, bowling, fishing, or just having plain fun." With group support, the person found comfort in discussing "how we used to do" and alternatives that included "having fun at a slower pace or engaging in less physically demanding activities." Financial problems from unemployment (even for those who have accumulated savings accounts); costs of medical treatments, transportation, and overnight stays; and continuing costs of normal household maintenance soon lead to depletion of funds. Such concerns create additional stress.

Some patients and families focus on problems relating to sexuality in the broader sense of the term, not just sex, but the loss of self-esteem, feelings of self-worth, body image, and dignity. Group members are encouraged to explore feelings of loneliness and love in relation to loss of sexuality. The support group provides the family member with opportunities to practice communication styles. Group members are encouraged to investigate the communication patterns they had prior to living with cancer and to practice open, honest communication patterns and true expression of feelings.

In conclusion, each function carried out by the oncologist, psychologist, and social worker is vital to approaching the patient as a total person. We have learned that patients and their family members frequently need to hear the relevant information provided by each member of the multidisciplinary team more than once. For this reason, arrangements are underway to videotape all 11 sessions of the oncology patient education series. These tapes will be added to our patient/family library. Videotapes present a distinct advantage for those patients who are unable to read due to educational or visual factors. Another videotape in preparation will introduce the ward staff (the oncologist, psychologist, social worker, head nurse, ward clerk, dietitian, etc.) to the patients. Being able to recognize familiar faces and names should increase comfort level and help to reduce fear or apprehension about the unknown.

THE TERMINAL PHASE: WORKING WITH THE DYING PATIENT

Variables impacting the patient's attitudes toward information and participation in medical decisions have been investigated (Cassileth et al. 1980) and especially warrant consideration in the terminal phase. The first major decision for the oncologist at this stage is to determine that attempts at either controlling or slowing the growth of tumor have failed and should be halted. This decision occurs when it is apparent that all active treatment options have failed, that any further chemotherapy would only be detrimental to the patient, worsening rather than enhancing quality of life and, perchance, hastening death. All treatment possibilities are reviewed carefully to determine if any viable options remain. When a decision is reached that no further measures can be taken to control disease, strictly palliative and comfort measures are then initiated. The treatment team, patient, and family are informed that the patient has reached the final stage of his disease. Whenever feasible, it is preferable to relay this crucial information to the patient in the company of his family or significant others. Phrasing is very important in softening the impact of this devastating news. It can be beneficial to combine the information that aggressive treatment is being stopped with the addition of a positive statement outlining the future course of action to be implemented. If the goal is pain control, then considerable time should be devoted to an explanation of the mechanisms that will be employed to achieve optimal pain control. Often it is necessary to alleviate fears about addiction to pain medication. The patient is given the opportunity to monitor pain control and request different types of pain medication depending on particular symptoms. Family members' help is solicited in this process. The goal is to make the transition as painless as possible as patients move from active treatment status to palliative/comfort care. The patient and family members become active participants to help achieve maximal comfort.

Concerns that frequently emerge at this phase involve the extent to which comfort measures extend life. For example, continuation of tube feedings does not "prolong the misery" in obviously terminal patients, but withdrawal of feedings upon which the family and patient place much value can be detrimental. Instead, patient and family are educated about problems to monitor in tube feedings, such as diarrhea, vomiting, and intolerance of feedings—all factors that influence patient comfort. Should any of these symptoms occur, tube feedings are stopped. Further, patients and family members learn about problems with infection that frequently occur in terminally ill cancer patients. Family members often express concern that antibiotics will prolong life. Although antibiotics may extend life only for days or hours, consideration must be given to the enhanced quality of life when confusion and agitation are prevented or reduced and debilitating fevers are controlled.

During the terminal stage, it is very important to establish physical contact while talking with patients. This physical contact is a vital nonverbal communication tool in the physician–patient relationship. The physician should sit, talk at eye level, hold the patient's hand, touch the patient's arm. Although difficult initially, a natural urge that is often smothered becomes a natural urge that is expressed, once the physician realizes how important it is to patients. The touch becomes a nonverbal communication of regret that nothing more can be done. While the touch expresses sympathy, words communicate what steps will be taken to promote physical comfort.

As long as the patient remains responsive, important communications are directed to him. Conferences with family members are held in the patient's room when feasible, but any patient request for a confidential session is honored. At this stage of the disease, patients may ask, "How long will I live?" When treatment options have been exhausted and it is obvious that the patient can survive only a limited amount of time—weeks or a few months—he or she should be informed if he or she requests the information. Direct questions require honest answers. Some patients, however, present this question in such a vague manner that it is clear no answers are desired. Reminders that estimations are not infallible can be presented through examples. A frequently used example is a patient whose treatment was ended and he was sent home to die 1 1/2 years ago. During his recent clinic appointment, he described plans for an upcoming fishing trip.

Another important aspect of care is a willingness to allow the patient to express whatever religious beliefs he may hold, and to share in that experience. Irrespective of the physician's personal beliefs, the terminal stage of illness is a time when patients can receive much comfort and courage from religion. Indeed, it can be a source of comfort for both patient and physician to share in that final stage of the patient's life and to offer it up to a higher power in the belief that He will handle everything. Such willingness to share is of great benefit in helping to maintain and enhance rapport between patient, family, and physician.

Life-threatening illnesses often mean that individuals must endure prolonged suffering and a lengthy process of dying. It is normal for feelings of helplessness and loss of control to be associated with this process. Some fear what must be endured prior to death. One elderly patient who was agitated and delirious remained lucid enough to communicate in his way that he was dying. His major issue was, "I just want to know how hard it is to die." Experiences on this cancer ward were shared with the patient, who learned that staff members were committed to maintaining patient comfort, so that patients died peacefully. The reassurance provided by the psychologist was then reinforced by the oncologist and nursing staff, who also told him they would make it as easy as possible for him to die. His agitation disappeared and he died peacefully a few days later. The most important point physicians must remember is to listen to their patients—listen with the eyes, the ears, and the heart—and the patients will tell them what is needed.

Achieving a level of comfort with one's own views of dying enables one to work more effectively with the patient's views about impending death and to communicate that death is an acceptable issue to confront in psychotherapy. A variety of opinions about dying will be encountered; for some, death is seen as providing peace and relief from suffering, as a "better place," and as a natural conclusion to life. One patient explained to his teenage children that everyone will die. He could be killed in a car accident and die tomorrow. The only difference for him was that he was fortunate enough to have his doctor tell him when death would come. Over the course of psychotherapy and disease progression, patients frequently change their goals, from hoping for a cure, to an extension of life, to praying to be able to walk as long as possible; from wanting three more years, to one year, to three months, to one more visit with family, to being thankful every morning when they awaken and have one more day. Some experience relief when they know that death is near because they are "tired of fighting." In the terminal stages of disease, patients desperately need to know that they will not be deserted.

Frequency of therapy sessions increases when death approaches. Patients who have struggled so hard in their battle against cancer need to have professionals communicate understanding about the reality of their endurance and demonstrate empathy for their profound emotional agony.

Another obstacle for patients is the difficulty of establishing relationships with other patients on the ward, then observing them decline and die. In a sense, "living" on a cancer ward, watching others grow more debilitated and die, forces one to deal with feelings about death and dying. Such experiences can challenge one's ability to cope with one's disease.

Sometimes, patients may live weeks or months beyond the time their medical condition should allow because, seemingly, they need to survive to help some family member prepare for their death. One of our recent younger patients was not expected to survive the night, but he managed to endure another 48 hours until his children, mother, and sisters could arrive to be with him and his wife and exchange their goodbyes. He allowed his family to share not only his agony, but also his courage and love.

It is remarkable how debilitated persons can complete their business. One patient whose wife had died from cancer several years ago worked through his grief over that loss, then proceeded to conduct his life review, resulting in a feeling of peace with himself and his life and impending death. He was able to look back and be grateful for the "good" years following his diagnosis, accepted the fact that his quality of life would not improve, and was ready to die after he had moved friends to that point. Just before he died, he winked and said, "It's a piece of cake." As another patient stated, "No one came to stay, we only came to visit."

Coping with loss of physical health, physical and emotional pain, loneliness, and separation from loved ones can hinder any human being's efforts to survive. It is often helpful to remind the patient of other "tough" times and to explore how the person survived them—combat experiences in World War II, loss of loved ones, and so on. Patients may be reminded that they are survivors and helped to call upon previous coping strategies. In such crisis situations, even a little improvement in terms of reducing distress can mean very much. Powerful emotions and grief can be very frightening for the older veteran with little understanding of psychiatric nomenclature or affective disorders. Such patients frequently say, "I am afraid I will start crying and not be able to stop . . ." This fear may well be based on World War II experiences when one in ten combat veterans was discharged for "combat fatigue." Traditional masculine stereotypes interfere with open expression of sadness and grief, but our patients help each other. One World War I veteran said during a support group meeting, "I cry; it provides a great sense of relief."

Losses associated with cancer frequently elicit memories of prior losses. The World War II combat veteran or POW may vividly reexperience that earlier pain. Sometimes World War II Post-traumatic Stress Disorders are evident for the first time. A patient may at last decide to deal with grief over the loss of a spouse several years before. Fear of abandonment may be a realistic concern during the terminal phase. Occasionally, families "run," but with staff support they generally are able to persevere. One patient was served divorce papers while hospitalized after his cancer surgery because his spouse did not want to be married to a cancer patient. Another patient's daughter requested that he stay away from her home because she did not want to catch his cancer. Too often, patients and families have to deal with feelings of rejection from family and friends; fortunately, many others describe increased support from others.

A family member shared that "Cancer is the only subject we cannot discuss." After investigation of past and current communication patterns, it was discovered that what could not be discussed was not cancer but their concerns and fears about the impending separation from their loved ones. Anticipatory grief is a painful experience. However, with the support of professional staff and the Caregivers Support Group, anticipatory grief work is done. Group members are encouraged to reminisce, to share events relative to their experiences with the terminally ill cancer patient. They are encouraged to acknowledge that anticipatory grief is painful. The group participates by listening with the heart and offering verbal and nonverbal messages of understanding.

The Oncology Caregivers Support Group provides a supportive field for family members to discuss and receive information regarding burial arrangements. Family members who are working through a grief process will sometimes initiate a request for information and support regarding the advantages or disadvantages of prearrangement of funerals and the V.A. policy for burial of patients who die in the V.A. Hospital. Valuable information can be gathered from some members who already have investigated burial arrangements. The family member who initiates discussion regarding burial will usually share with the group that the purpose of thinking of or actually prearranging a funeral is "to get on with the business of living." The patient has the advantage of knowing that his or her surviving relatives will not have to face that planning alone.

On occasion the social worker will rehearse with the family member the V.A. procedures at the time of the patient's death. The social worker informs the family member of the possible questions, such as the name of the funeral home, the patient's parents' full names, request for an autopsy, and questions about widow's benefits. The family member is made aware that similar questions will be asked by a person other than the social worker at the time of death. (It is interesting to note that most caregivers have difficulty remembering full names of patient's parents.) Family members receiving this information share that they feel "partially prepared," at least knowing what will be expected.

The clinical social worker frequently witnesses the patient's death with the family members. Witnessing the death of a loved one is one of the most difficult tasks anyone can face. Bereavement counseling—being of comfort—is a ministry of love and a most rewarding experience. A few basic principles of bereavement counseling are: be sincere—think how you would want to be supported; listen with the heart rather than with the head, permitting grief and sorrow to surface; allow those who are mourning to express grief without being judgmental; be available to the caregiver throughout the bereavement process.

As a result of patient and family support and education, through individual patient contacts and involvement in educational and support group sessions, there can be an improvement in patient/family relationships; increased family support; decreased patient/family stress while adapting to cancer, the ward routine, and the treatment plan; and informed patients and family members actively involved in the treatment plan. Family members are observed providing emotional support for each other during crisis periods. They share coping techniques; they make plans to provide continued support by phone and letter. Consequently family members feel less alone.

The Oncology Family Reunion concept was created to continue our bond of love and shared experiences. The yearly Reunion, first held in June, 1984, is organized to involve all current patients and families, as well as families of deceased patients. Each year since its organization the attendance has increased. Many emotions are shared, especially feelings of "we care." Family members and patients have expressed their enjoyment of the reunion events by writing letters to staff and telling us in conversations from one year to the next, "I hope the reunion idea will never cease." It is not always possible for some family members to attend, but even they are reminded that they are not forgotten. Indeed, a support group for surviving significant others has been established to allow continued resolution of grief work.

The process of providing education and support for terminally ill patients and their families contributes to the development of staff resources. One can witness raw courage and sheer inner strength while sharing the ordeals in the lives of dying cancer patients. The horrifying circumstances patients often have to endure to continue living gives new meaning to the phrase "struggling to live." Sharing a patient's fight for each breath of life, and the sacrifices patients are willing to make in order to maintain life, certainly enhances one's consciousness of life's preciousness. Understanding and appreciation of these personal challenges will enhance the effectiveness of service providers.

Staff attitudes have a powerful impact on patients and their families. The words of Fr. Nouwen (1974) describe the atmosphere we strive to maintain on our oncology ward:

> When we honestly ask ourselves which persons in our lives mean the most to us, we often find that it is those who, instead of giving much advice, solutions, or cures, have chosen rather to share our pain and touch our wounds with a gentle and tender hand. The friend who can be silent with us in a moment of despair or confusion, who can stay with us in an hour of grief and bereavement, who can tolerate not knowing, not curing, not healing, and face with us the reality of our powerlessness, that is the friend who cares.

REFERENCES

ANDERSON, B. L. 1985. "Sexual Function and Morbidity Among Cancer Survivors: Current Status and Future Research Directions." *Cancer* 55:1835–1842.

CASSEL, E. 1985. *Talking with Patients.* Cambridge, MA: MIT Press.

CASSILETH, B. R., R. M. HEIBERGER, V. MARCH, AND K. SUTTON-SMITH. 1982. "Effect of Audiovisual Cancer Programs on Patients and Families. *Journal of Medical Education* 57:54–59.

CASSILETH, B. R., R. V. ZUPKIS, K. SUTTON-SMITH, V. MARCH. 1980. "Information and Participation Preferences Among Cancer Patients." *Annals of Internal Medicine* 92:832–836.

CRAIG, T. J. AND M. D. ABELOFF. 1974. Psychiatric Symptomatology Among Hospitalized Cancer Patients." *American Journal of Psychiatry* 131:1323–1327.

DEROGATIS, L. R., M. FELDSTEIN, G. MORROW, A. SCHMALE, M. SCHMITT, C. GATES, B. MURAWSKI, J. HOLLAND, D. PENMAN, N. MELISARATOS, A. J. EXELOW, AND L. M. ADLER. 1979. "A Survey of Psychotropic Drug Prescriptions in an Oncology Population." *Cancer* 44(5):1919–1929.

DEROGATIS, L. R., G. R. MORROW, J. FETTING, D. PENMAN, S. PIASETSKY, A. M. SCHMALE, M. HENRICHS, AND C. L. CARNICKE JR. 1983. "The Prevalence of Psychiatric Disorders Among Cancer Patients." *Journal of the American Medical Association* 249(6):751–757.

GOLDBERG, R. J. 1981. "Management of Depression in the Patient with Advanced Cancer." *Journal of the American Medical Association* 246:373–376.

GORDON, W. A., I. FREIDENBERGS, L. DILLER, M. HIBBARD, C. WOLF, L. LEVINE, R. LIPKINS, O. EZRACHI, AND D. LUCIDO. 1980. "Efficacy of Psychosocial Intervention with Cancer Patients." *Journal of Consulting Clinical Psychology* 48(6):743–759.

HERSH, S. P. 1985. "Psychologic Aspects of Patients with Cancer." In V. DeVity Jr., S. Hellman, and S. Rosenberg, eds. *Cancer: Principles and Practices of Oncology.* Philadelphia: Lippincott, p. 55.

HERZOFF, N. E. 1979. "A Therapeutic Group for Cancer Patients and Their Families." *Cancer Nursing* 2:469–474.

JOHNSON, J. 1982. "The Effects of a Patient Education Course on Persons with a Chronic Illness." *Cancer Nursing* 5:117–123.

KUBLER-ROSS, E. 1978. *To Live Until We Say Good-bye.* Englewood Cliffs, NJ: Prentice-Hall.

LAUER, P., S. P. MURPHY, AND M. J. POWERS. 1892. "Needs of Cancer Patients: A Comparison of Nurse and Patient Perceptions." *Nursing Research* 31:11–16.

NOUWEN, H. J. M. 1974. *Out of Solitude.* Notre Dame: Ave Marie Press.

PLUMB, M. M. AND J. HOLLAND. 1977. "Comparative Studies of Psychological Function in Patients with Advanced Cancer." *Journal of Psychosomatic Medicine* 39:264–276.

SCHIPPER, H., J. CLINCH, A. MCMURRAY, AND M. LEVITT. 1984. "Measuring the Quality of Life of Cancer Patients: The Functional Living Index—Cancer: Its Development and Validation." *Journal of Clinical Oncology* 2:472–483.

SPITZER, W. O., A. J. DOBSON, J. HALL, ET AL. 1981. "Measuring the Quality of Life of Cancer Patients: A Concise QL-Index for Use by Physicians." *Journal of Chronic Diseases* 34:585–597.

STEWART, B. E., B. E. MEYEROWITZ, L. E. JACKSON, K. L. YARKIN, AND J. H. HARVEY. 1982. "Psychological Stress Associated with Outpatient Oncology Nursing." *Cancer Nursing* 5:383–387.

WEISMAN, A. D. 1972. *On Dying and Denying.* New York: Human Sciences Press.

WEISMAN, A. D. 1976. "Early Diagnosis of Vulnerability in Cancer Patients." *American Journal of Medical Science* 271:187–196.

WEISMAN, A. D. AND J. W. WORDEN. 1975. "Psychosocial Analysis of Cancer Deaths." *Omega* 6:61–75.

WELCH-MCCAFFREY, D. 1983. "When It comes to Cancer—Think Family." *Nursing* 13:32–35.

WORDEN, J. W. AND WEISMAN, A. D. 1980. "Do Cancer Patients Really Want Counseling?" *General Hospital Psychiatry* 2:100–103.

2

The Caring Process and the Cancer Patient

Joan Paternoster, RN, MS

Caring is a process essential to the growth, development, and survival of human beings (Gaylin 1976). Most health care professionals consider themselves to be caring individuals and are usually perceived that way by consumers of professional services. When consumers complain that health care providers do not care for and about them, it is generally believed that the fault lies with the professional. This may not be the case. The problem may arise due to a poor fit between the immediate needs of the client and the behaviors of the provider. The person with cancer has many different needs that surface at various times during the course of the disease and its treatment. Health care providers must be aware of the person's need level and demonstrate corresponding behaviors in order to communicate caring to the client.

This chapter discusses the process of caring as described in the social science and health care literature. The affective and task dimensions of the caring process are explicated. The relationship between need level and perception of caring is explored with application to persons with cancer.

THE CARING PROCESS

Caring is a process that has been described by philosophers and psychologists for many years but has only recently been identified as an area for research in the health sciences. The major non-health related writings on caring are found in the fields of philosophy and psychology. Mayeroff (1971), Buber (1958), May (1969) and Gaylin (1976), for example, write of the caring process or relationship and its contribution to the welfare of mankind.

According to the philosopher Mayeroff (1971), caring is an interpersonal

18

process that is undertaken with the intent of helping a person grow. In Mayeroff's schemata, caring is a reciprocal process related to the needs of the recipient, who remains independent from the caregiver. Responsibilities evolving from a caring relationship are willingly accepted by the caregiver. Caring involves devotion, which Mayeroff defined as congruence between what the caregivers want to do and what they feel they are supposed to do.

Buber (1958), also a philosopher, spoke of caring in the "I-Thou" relationship. He identified the "I-Thou" relationship as a realm in which one individual as subject recognizes, knows, and cares for another as subject. Each person in the relationship recognizes the other as a unique and valued being with whom he or she shares existence. Care is an essential component of the relationship that is manifest in the interaction between the participants.

In 1969 Rollo May, a psychologist, addressed caring in the therapeutic relationship. He said that care brings love and will together; it involves doing something about a situation. Care is a certain type of intentionality that requires a belief, on the part of the therapist, that what happens to the client matters. May identified the role of caring in the quality of life when he said, "Life comes from physical survival; but the good life comes from what we care about" (p. 286).

Gaylin (1976), a behavioral psychologist, described caring as rooted in man's biological nature. He believed that caring is unique to man and essential for survival. Gaylin's work centered on the mother–child relationship, but he acknowledged the existence of elements of caring in other relationships. Caring refers to a specific kind of love that enables a child to develop the capacity to love. Gaylin defined caring when he said, "To be cared for refers to all aspects of that word; to be taken care of, to be concerned about, to be worried over, to be supervised, to be attended to, to be loved" (p. 68).

Literature from the fields of psychology and philosophy speaks to caring in both personal and professional relationships and provides descriptions and definitions related to the process. Mayeroff (1971) and Buber (1958) saw caring as a process of growth and addressed the affective components. May (1969) and Gaylin (1976) took the process one step further by introducing the action component of caring in respect to the "doing for" or "doing something about" an individual's situation. They also spoke to the role of caring in the quality of life.

The health care literature related to caring is found primarily in the work of nursing. In recent years, nurses have studied the caring process in detail in an attempt not only to define and describe (Gaut 1983; Henry 1975; Leininger 1981, 1984) but also to quantify (Brown 1982; Larson 1984) the construct. Reported studies have been done from ethnographic, philosophical, phenomenological, and empirical perspectives.

Nurses' interest in caring stems from an American Nurses Association position paper published in 1965. That paper identified care as an essential component of nursing and delineated two components of caring in the following statement, "the care aspect is more than 'to take care of,' it is 'caring for' and 'caring about' as well" (p. 107). Definition and delineation of these action components has been the focus of nurses' research on caring.

Leininger (1984) who studied caring from an ethnographic perspective, believed care is the "hidden quality of human services that makes people satisfied or unsatisfied with health care services" (p. 8). Leininger discussed care in relation to cure and said that without care, cure cannot occur.

In 1975, Henry conducted a qualitative study that attempted to ascertain and describe the behaviors of nurses identified by patients as indicators of care. She interviewed 50 patients in a community setting and identified three major categories: (1) what the nurse does, (2) how the nurse does, and (3) how much the nurse does. This was the first study to identify two types of caring behaviors—task and affective. Henry concluded that caring requires both technical competence and interpersonal skills.

Gaut (1983), in a philosophical analysis of caring, attempted to understand what must be true in order to say that one person is caring for another. She determined that, in order to act in a caring capacity, the caregiver must have a knowledge of the person's situation and of the things that can be done to improve the situation, and choose and implement an action with the purpose of positively affecting the situation; the change must be judged on what is good for the person receiving care. In this analysis, Gaut makes a distinction between "caring for" and "caring about" an individual. She says that "caring for" involves providing for or being responsible for another while "caring about" implies a valuing of the other. Gaut believes that the "care about" dimension brings quality to the caring relationship. The " 'caring about' eliminates the apathy, indifference, obligation, withdrawal, isolation, manipulation, and possession in the one way relationships of 'caring for' in the limited sense of 'providing for' " (p. 316).

Recent studies have attempted to differentiate and define the two dimensions (Brown 1982; Larson 1984). In a study of hospitalized patients conducted in 1981, Brown sought to "identify, describe, and classify nursing behaviors perceived by patients as indicators of care" and "to examine the task and affective dimensions of care"(p. iii). Her study further validated Henry's findings that there are two dimensions of caring. Brown concluded that the caring experience involves an interaction between the client and the nurse; the task dimension is fundamental to caring but the affective dimension is also important. She described the interaction of the components in the caring process in the following statement: "The experience of being cared for by a nurse as described by the patients in the study is, indeed, made up of the qualities of the nurse's being that are expressed in the doing for and to the client'' (p. 147).

In an additional study undertaken in 1981, Larson looked at nurses' and patients' perceptions of important nurse caring behaviors. Her subjects were nurses and patients on inpatient oncology units. She measured six scales: (1) accessible, (2) explains and facilitates, (3) comforts, (4) anticipates, (5) trusting relationship, and (6) monitors and follows through. The patients in Larson's study were drawn from an inpatient hospital unit and were receiving active treatment for their disease. Larson found that there was incongruity between nurses' and patients' perception of caring behaviors, with nurses focusing on the affective areas of the ''comfort'' and ''trust'' domains and patients on the task areas of the ''monitors and follows through'' and ''accessibility'' domains. This study raises the question of the role of patients needing high-tech physical care in their perception of caring behaviors. Did the patients in this study value the task dimension of caring because they were at a specific need level?

Diers (1984), in discussing caring as a component of professionalism, said that caring is difficult and must be titrated to meet individual client needs. She made a distinction between thoughtful and planned care and tender loving care. Thoughtful and planned care is good care, but it must also be tender and loving to be quality care. Good care is basic to quality care; quality is not provided in isolation from technical skill. Together the components bring professionalization to practice.

Recent studies on caring have focused on the caring process and have identified two dimensions of care. These have been labeled as the ''task'' and the ''affective'' components (Brown 1982; Larson 1981). These seem to be analogous to the ''care for'' and ''care about'' dimensions of the caring process described by Gaut (1983). ''Care for'' refers to the tasks involved in providing for or being responsible for another while ''care about'' refers to an affective valuing and brings quality to the caring process.

The social science and health care literature provides a picture of caring as a process that consists of affective and task dimensions. The task dimension consists of actions related to the technical skills of the professional, while the affective dimension refers to the way in which the professional relates to the client in the interaction (ANA 1965; Brown, 1982; Gaylin 1976; Gaut 1983; Henry 1975; Larson 1984). The two components are hierarchical in nature, with the task dimension being basic to the affective dimension. The professional must be able to provide the ''care for'' or good care, or he can not be perceived of as providing the ''care about'' or quality component (Brown 1981; Diers 1984; Mayeroff 1971). Caring is an interpersonal process that is related to the client's needs and results in the improvement of the client's welfare (Gaut 1983; Mayeroff 1971).

MASLOW'S MOTIVATIONAL NEED THEORY

Abraham Maslow (1970) identified six needs that motivate a person's behavior. These needs are hierarchical in order and dominance as follows: (1) physiological, (2) safety, (3) love and belonging, (4) esteem and recognition, (5) self-actualization, and (6) aesthetic. In order to advance to a higher level of need, all needs of lower order must be at least partially fulfilled. Needs may overlap, but new higher level needs will not emerge until lower level needs are at least partially fulfilled.

Physiological needs for water, food, oxygen, sleep, and sex (in the physiological sense) are basic for humans. If these needs are unmet, a person will be hungry, thirsty, anxious, and frustrated, and conflict will arise. The second need is for safety, feelings of physical security, order and stability. Unmet safety needs are manifested in separation anxiety, physical harm, and pain. The third level need is for love and belonging, which includes affiliation, acceptance, and companionship. Persons who are experiencing unmet emergent love and belonging needs will be lonely and alienated. The fourth need is for esteem and recognition, which includes both self-esteem and esteem of others. Inability to meet esteem needs will result in feelings of helplessness, inferiority, and worthlessness. The fifth level need is for self-actualization, the experience of self-fulfillment. Persons who never self-actualize will have chronic feelings of inferiority. Aesthetic needs, the sixth level, are manifested in a desire for beauty, truth, order, and harmony (Maslow 1970).

Maslow's needs are sometimes also grouped into primary or survival needs and secondary or ego needs. In this orientation, the physiological needs are considered to be the primary needs, with all others seen as secondary needs (Mitchell 1977; Peplau 1952), although there may be some overlap at the safety level. If an individual has fears for personal security and bodily integrity or is in physical pain, that may be a survival need or a combination of survival and ego, rather than purely an ego need.

RELATIONSHIP OF THE CARING PROCESS AND MOTIVATIONAL NEED LEVEL

It can be seen from the foregoing discussion that the caring process and need level have some commonalities and some differences. They are both behaviorally and verbally expressed, hierarchical in nature, and can be delineated into two discrete entities. Source of origin and purpose are points of difference. The two concepts appear to be complementary and can be utilized together by the health care professional.

Individuals express their needs through behaviors that are observable to caregivers, such as hunger, frustration, alienation, and fear, and by verbalization of feelings of helplessness, lack of confidence, and disharmony. Caregivers communicate caring by behaviors such as providing food and touching that seek to meet individuals' physical and emotional needs, by verbalizing interest and concern for their welfare, and by willingly accepting the responsibilities involved in the caring relationship.

An individual's needs are hierarchical in that lower-level needs emerge first and must be satisfied before higher-level needs emerge. For example, the person who is hungry will be motivated to seek food even in the face of physical danger. Perceptions of caring behavior appear similarly hierarchical. Both the task and affective components were identified in all groups studied, but the task dimension seems to be fundamental to the affective dimension (Brown 1981; Larson, 1984).

Maslow (1970) originally described motivational needs as six discrete entities, but they can also be grouped into two categories: primary or physiological needs and secondary or ego needs (Peplau 1952). These are consistent with the two dimensions of caring described in the social science literature and validated by health care researchers.

Motivational needs and caring are grounded in different sources and serve different purposes. Needs originate within the individual and motivate him to behave in ways that will lead to need fulfillment. The individual is constantly striving to fulfill emergent needs and to move to a higher level of function. Needs arise within the individual and can only be expressed by the individual experiencing them. Caring is an interpersonal process that requires both a caregiver and a care recipient and can only be validated within the relationship. Needs arise from distress and motivate an individual to behave in ways that will satisfy the need and relieve the tension (Peplau 1952). Caring is an interpersonal process that facilitates the satisfaction of needs and relief of stress and tension.

The concepts of motivational need and caring can be seen as having a complementary relationship: as need level rises from primary to secondary, appropriate caring behaviors rise from task to affective. For example, the individual who has many physiological needs will probably perceive the caring professional as one who has the skills to meet those needs. Similarly, the individual with high needs for love and belonging will respond to the person or group who exhibits more affective behaviors. This is supported by studies conducted in inpatient settings that showed subjects with high-tech needs rating the task component of caring higher than the affective component (Larson 1984), and those in community settings with low-tech needs rating the affective component higher than the task component (Henry 1975). Need levels are not static; they change with physical and psychological status. Perceptions of caring behaviors can also be expected to change with shifts in motivational needs.

Therefore, in order to facilitate the process of need fulfillment, the caregiver must fit the caring behavior to the emergent need of the care recipient.

IMPLICATIONS FOR THE PERSON WITH CANCER

Cancer is a multifaceted disease that manifests in many ways. Target organs, treatment modalities, and prognosis differ according to medical diagnosis. The progress of the disease is difficult to project and may vary with each individual. Some persons progress in a direct line from diagnosis through treatment to cure, remission, or death. Others may be in and out of remission for years. Treatment may be one dimensional or multidimensional. Persons with cancer can be expected to move up and down the need levels and therefore will require variance in caring behaviors. For example, the person who has just received a diagnosis of cancer will probably be motivated by safety and/or love and belonging needs and respond to affective caring behaviors. The same person when undergoing active chemotherapy will have high physiological needs and be responsive to the caregiver who possesses the technical skills that will facilitate the treatment.

The professional working with the person with cancer must be aware of the emergent need level of the care recipient and adjust caring behaviors to complement those needs. The caregiver must also be aware of his own caring style and the expertise that he has to offer the client. Since a professional can not be all things to all clients, it may be necessary, at least temporarily, to defer to another caregiver who best meets the client's emergent needs.

REFERENCES

AMERICAN NURSES ASSOCIATION. 1965. *A Position Paper*. New York: American Nurses Association.

BROWN, L. 1982. "Behaviors of Nurses Perceived by Hospitalized Patients as Indicators of Care." Doctoral Dissertation, University of Colorado, Boulder. *Dissertation Abstracts International* 43:11B.

BUBER, M. 1958. *I and Thou*. New York: Scribner.

DIERS, D. 1984. "To Profess—To Be a Profession." *Journal of the New York State Nurses Association* 15:22–29.

GAUT, D. 1983. "Development of a Theoretically Accurate Description of Caring." *Western Journal of Nursing Research* 5:313–324.

GAYLIN, W. 1976. *Caring*. New York: Alfred A. Knopf.

HENRY, O. 1975. "Nurse Behaviors Perceived by Patients as Indicators of Caring." Doctoral Dissertation, Catholic University, Washington, D.C. *Dissertation Abstracts International* 36: 02B.

LARSON, P. 1984. "Important Nurse Caring Behaviors Perceived by Patients with Cancer." *Oncology Nursing Forum* 11(6):46–50.

LARSON, P. 1981. "Oncology Patients' and Professional Nurses' Perceptions of Important Nurse

Caring Behaviors." Doctoral Dissertation, University of California, San Francisco. *Dissertation Abstracts International* 42:02B.

LEININGER, M. 1984. "Care: The Essence of Nursing and Health." In *Care: The Essence of Nursing and Health.* Thorofare, NJ: Slack, pp. 3–15.

LEININGER, M. 1981. "The Phenomenon of Caring: Importance, Research Questions and Theoretical Considerations." In *Caring: An Essential Human Need.* Thorofare, NJ: Slack, pp. 3–15.

MASLOW, A. 1970. *Motivation and Personality,* Second Edition. New York: Harper and Row.

MAY, R. 1969. *Love and Will.* New York: Dell.

MAYEROFF, M. 1971. *On Caring.* New York: Harper and Row.

MITCHELL, P. 1977. *Concepts Basic to Nursing.* New York: McGraw-Hill.

PEPLAU, H. 1952. *Interpersonal Relations in Nursing.* New York: Putnam.

ADDITIONAL READING

UNITED STATES DEPARTMENT OF HEALTH AND HUMAN SERVICES, NATIONAL CANCER INSTITUTE. 1980. *Coping with Cancer: A Resource for the Health Professional* (Publication L80–2080). Washington, D.C.: National Institutes of Health.

3

Factors That Contribute to Control and Hopefulness

Barbara R. Breitbart, PhD

In this chapter, I will discuss the concept of taking control of one's illness as a mediating factor in reducing stress, depression, and helplessness, as well as enhancing a sense of hopefulness. I will also discuss the relationship of mind to health and disease, and how the body seems to have a way of following the mind's expectations.

Most current thinking about the mechanisms that link psychosocial stimuli to physical disorders in some way invoke stress as a factor that precipitates illness and influences its course and outcome. If a person is suffering from a life-threatening disease, he or she is most likely also suffering from severe emotional stress. Patients' emotional reactions to their illness, along with their available coping responses, influence for better or worse the course and outcome of the disease.

There is increasing evidence that a number of different psychological processes mediate or modify the link between stress and illness. This evidence is so clear that it is inappropriate to assess the effects of stress on disease without considering the patients' coping mechanisms as one important mediating variable.

When a traumatic event first occurs, as when one learns he has cancer, it arouses a heightened state of emotion best described as fear or panic. The person is thrown into a reactive phase, characterized by automatic emotional reactions. Attempts at adaptation follow. If the patient can reduce the trauma through some coping mechanism, fear will be reduced; if he or she cannot, fear will be replaced with depression, a state of helplessness will ensue, and this psychological distress may be translated directly into a physiologal response. Psychological factors do not influence disease in some mystic fashion. Rather,

26

the physiological status of the host is altered in some way. Numerous studies, in both animals and humans, clearly demonstrate this.

In one experiment (Weiss 1968), a rat was exposed to an electric shock which it could avoid or escape by touching its nose to a panel. A second rat was given exactly the same shocks, but could not escape or avoid them. In other words, the yoked control rat had no control over the shocks. Thus, the two animals received exactly the same physical stressor; they differed only in their control over the shock.

In these circumstances, if a difference in pathology as manifested by the development of gastric lesions was observed between the two rats, the difference could not be due to the physical stressor, which was the same for both subjects, but must be due to the psychological difference inherent in having control over the stressor, as compared with being helpless. The animals that were able to avoid or escape shock developed fewer gastric lesions than their helpless counterparts.

In a similar experiment closer to our topic, and using the same yoked paradigm, three groups of rats were injected with live tumor cells. One day later, two of the three groups were subjected to electric shock; one group could avoid or escape the shock and the other could not. A control group received no shocks. The results showed that 73 percent of the helpless rats developed cancer, while only 37 percent of the rats that could control the shock by escape developed cancer. There was no significant difference between the group that could control shock and the control group, which received no shocks. (Visintainer et al. 1982).

Clearly, stress *per se* does not appear to be the critical feature that led to these physiological changes, but rather the organism's inability to cope behaviorally in a stress situation over which it has no control.

In looking for links between coping and disease processes, the assumption is often made that individuals who utilize maladaptive coping styles will become anxious, depressed, and helpless. These negative feelings may be reflected in further distress, leading to decreases in bodily resistance and exacerbation of the disease.

Research with both animals and humans has suggested that the greater the perceived controllability of a stressor, the less harmful are its effects on the organism. Being able to control a noxious event, believing that one can control the event, or perceiving that one can control other aspects of the environment can reduce the impact of a stressful event.

When individuals encounter aversive events over which they perceive little or no control, a state of helplessness ensues (Seligman 1975). The psychological state of helplessness undermines response initiation along with its adaptive behavioral repertoire. The state is characterized by passive behavior, negative expectations and hopelessness. Control, whether real or perceived, appears to mediate the effects of helplessness. Any activity that diminishes helplessness will contribute to the patient's sense of control.

A study was performed at the National Cancer Institute on a group of patients who had been operated on for malignant melanoma, with apparently successful results. The study revealed that relapse did not tend to occur among those patients who confronted their illness with an active, positive approach.

An active, positive approach involves choice and information seeking. People who have dealt successfully with serious illness comment on the need to make decisions regarding their illness. They seek out information, they are assertive, and they persist when they believe their needs and requirements are being overlooked. These are the patients some physicians consider difficult or uncooperative, but these are also the patients who are most likely to get well. In a study of 35 women with metastatic breast cancer, it was found that long-term survivors had poor relationships with their physicians as judged by the physicians (Derogatis as reported by Seigel 1986). Researchers at the National Cancer Institute also found that aggressive, "bad" patients tend to have more killer T cells than docile, "good" patients (reported in Seigel 1986). The very process of actively moving toward participating in treatment helps to reinforce the sense of control and personal direction that cancer so typically impairs. The health care team should avoid placing their patients in a passive, dependent position. By giving patients the opportunity to exercise some form of control over their therapy and environment, we as health professionals can help the patient to learn active ways of being and doing that will enhance their sense of control and contribute to a state of hopefulness rather than helplessness.

With self-management procedures, the therapist can teach patients to change aspects of their environment; the passive role of the patient is then transformed into the active role of the participant. The role of the therapist becomes one of devising effective behavior-change techniques and of motivating the patient to carry them out.

To become active participants, patients need information regarding their illness, treatment, and home health care. The sense of mastery engendered by knowledge increases a sense of personal control and minimizes the sense of helplessness.

One study reported that giving a group of cancer patients all the facts about their illness resulted in considerably less depression, with a resultant decrease in the use of psychotropic drugs, compared with a group given little or no information (Gerla et al. 1960).

Nutritional and dietary changes not only offer patients a chance to participate in their own treatment, but also engender a sense of hopefulness. When patients are encouraged to participate actively, they are able to move from an initial helpless position to a new-found ability to work actively and constructively toward health.

Self-regulatory strategies such as visual imagery, autogenic training, biofeedback, and relaxation techniques, in addition to their primary role as stress reduction techniques, help toward contributing a sense of control as well as a sense of hopefulness. Simonton et al. (1978), using these techniques, reported increased survival rates in cancer patients who have embarked on such programs.

How effective are spiritual and alternative forms of healing? Cases of so-called spontaneous regression of cancer may be instructive. Several case histories (Everson and Cole 1966) report that regression of tumors coincided with treatments as diverse as prayer, conversion to Christian Science, mud packs, vitamin therapy, and force feeding.

Physicians in the past who favored such modalities as bleeding, purging through emetics, and physical contact with unicorn horns or powdered mummies no doubt regarded their techniques as efficacious. Today, we recognize that whatever efficacy these treatments had was most probably related to the faith placed in them by both patient and physician, and their concomitant expectations.

The point is that the belief system of the patient is sometimes a key factor in the healing force, so that what a person believes will happen with his disease and treatment may be related to the course and outcome.

In one case history, Klopfer (1957) described a patient with very advanced lymphosarcoma who begged to be treated with Krebiozen, after he had learned of a number of fantastic cures with this new chemical from Germany. After the patient's initial series of treatments, his tumor masses "melted like snowballs on a hot stove." Where previously he had required an oxygen mask merely to sustain himself during daily activities, he was now able to fly a plane at 12,000 feet without any effort. He continued to do well, but following some unfavorable publicity suggesting that Krebiozen was ineffective, he again became bedridden. In desperation, his physician told him that the adverse reports were not accurate and had been based on faulty preparations of the drug. He indicated that he now had available a supply of a fresher active potent principle, which the patient eagerly accepted. He was actually given distilled water, and once again the disease disappeared rapidly with clinical remission. Subsequently it was announced that the Food and Drug Administration and the American Medical Association had found Krebiozen to be worthless. Following this report, the patient succumbed to his disease within a matter of days.

This anecdote should put a lie to the myth, still prevalent among some members of the scientific community, that if a patient responds to a placebo, his symptoms must be either imagined or feigned. More importantly, we should learn from this case history and many others like it that if the patient has faith in a procedure and believes in its effectiveness—whether it be laetrile, macrobiotics, megavitamins, meditation, or visual imagery—the body seems able to utilize that belief, which manifests itself as a healing force. Therefore, any of these methods can be valuable adjuncts (not substitutes) for the standard medical treatment program, whether they are efficacious in themselves or not.

It has been said that the history of medical treatment until relatively recently is the history of the placebo effect. That the body possesses awesome capabilities to effect changes induced by psychological factors seems clear. What we need is a clearer understanding of how placebos exert their effects, both positively and negatively.

The bulk of medical literature on placebos treat the placebo effect as a nuisance variable, worthy of notice only for the disruption it can cause upon inadequately designed experiments. One hears, for example, that psychotherapy will become a more potent tool when it is isolated from the concomitant placebo effect. It is my belief that these same psychological factors that are eschewed as artifacts in most research constitute legitimate and effective treatments, worthy of exploration and exploitation as therapeutic interventions in their own right. The nature of placebos and the responses they can evoke are intriguing, because they point to the existence of an innate healing ability. The common thread is the power of belief. Placebos can relieve pain, they can induce sleep or mental alertness, they can bring about dramatic remissions in both symptoms and objective signs of disease, and so forth. By the same token, they can elicit negative outcomes, including nausea, skin rashes, serious allergic reactions, damage to organs, and even death. Thus, physical processes may respond to beliefs involving both positive and negative expectations. The positive expectations result in a state of hopefulness, which enhances the will to live, along with its concomitant beneficial physiologic effects. As Norman Cousins wrote in *Anatomy of an Illness* (1979), "The will to live is not a theoretical abstraction, but a physiologic reality with therapeutic characteristics." Negative expectations, on the other hand, result in a state of hopelessness, which is akin to passive suicide. I'm not suggesting a regression to primitive medicine, but rather that we become open and receptive to possibilities not yet understood by science.

Nor am I advocating patient deception by the use of placebos. The placebo effect can be elicited by nondeceptive means in which the use of a placebo need not be resorted to. In other words, the use of a placebo and the placebo effect can be differentiated. For example, a woman of Christian Science faith failed to heal after surgery to correct retinal detachment, despite the relative simplicity of the procedure. Afterwards, she indicated to the surgeon that having surgery was in conflict with her Christian Science beliefs. Before reoperating, the surgeon made clear to her that he was only doing a mechanical task akin to realigning a broken bone, and that her faith was the major factor in healing. His statement helped her to reconcile her Christian Science beliefs with the necessity of surgery and she healed quickly after the second operation (Mason 1969).

As this vignette suggests, if the emotional needs of the patient are not met, even the active medical treatment may fall short of its mark.

By providing an atmosphere of hope, faith, and confidence, the health care team can, at the very least, enhance the therapeutic value of the medical treatment, so that patients respond to a treatment regimen not with despair and hopelessness but with a mood of challenge and hope. In the Simonton book *Getting Well Again* (1978), there is a sentence that reads, "In the face of uncertainty, there is nothing wrong with hope. Refusal to hope is akin to a decision to die." I'm not referring to false hope.

We can provide patients with realistic underpinnings for their hopes by reviewing with them actual cases as severe as or more severe than their own, in which the patients came through and now live useful and productive lives. Physicians can also persuade their patients that although there are no guarantees, they have a real chance so long as both patient and physician give it their best efforts. The existence of resources such as hope and confidence contribute to a sense of retaining control and are potentially potent therapeutic factors.

If patients are encouraged to believe there is more to medicine than pills and incisions, we will help to give credence to the idea that they can exercise some influence over the course and outcome of their disease. The quality of mind is no less important than the quality of medical treatment.

REFERENCES

COUSINS, N. 1979. *Anatomy of an Illness as Perceived by the Patient.* New York: W. W. Norton.

EVERSON, T. C. AND W. H. COLE. 1966. *Spontaneous Regression of Cancers.* Philadelphia: W. B. Saunders.

GERLE, B., G. LUNDEN, AND D. SANDBLOM. 1960. "The Patient with Inoperable Cancer from the Psychiatric and Social Standpoint." *Cancer* 13:1206–1217.

KLOPFER, B. 1957. "Psychological Variables in Human Cancer." *Journal of Projective Techniques* 21:331–340.

MASON, R. C., G. CLARK, R. B. REEVS, AND S. B. WAGNER. 1969. "Acceptance and Healing." *Journal of Religion and Health* 8:123–142.

SEIGEL, B. S. 1986. *Love, Medicine and Miracles.* New York: Harper and Row.

SELIGMAN, M. E. 1975. *Helplessness: On Depression Development and Death.* San Francisco: W. H. Freeman and Co.

SIMONTON, O. C., S. MATTHEWS-SIMONTON, AND J. CREIGHTON. 1978. *Getting Well Again: A Step-By-Step Self-Help Guide to Overcoming Cancer for Patients and Their Families.* Los Angeles: Jeremy P. Tarcher.

STAVRAKY, R. B., C. N. BUCK, J. S. LOTT, AND J. M WANKLIN. 1968. "Psychological Factors in the Outcome of Human Cancer." *Journal of Psychosomatic Research* 12:251–259.

VISINTAINER, M. A., J. R. VOLPICELLI, AND M. E. B. SELIGMAN. 1982. "Tumor Rejection in Rats after Inescapable or Escapable Shock." *Sciences* 216:437–439.

WEISS, J. 1968. "Effects of Coping Responses on Stress." *Journal of Comparative and Physiological Psychology* 65(2):251–260.

ADDITIONAL READING

BROWN, F. 1966. "The Relationship Between Cancer and Personality." *Annals of the New York Academy of Sciences* 125:865–873.

4

Symptom Control, Ethics, and Communication Patterns: Crucial Topics in Cancer Education

Samuel C. Klagsbrun, MD

TRAINING IN SYMPTOM CONTROL

Symptom control is not a separate subject in medical, nursing, or social work schools. It is a subject that is subsumed under other headings for other purposes. If one were to list the major care issues, especially, for example, in terminal illness resulting from cancer, one would have to put symptom control at the top of the list. Yet there is no place in the medical school curriculum where it is addressed as a specialty area. There should be a place for it in pharmacology and in internal medicine. The topics of narcotic addiction and pain control are subsumed under pharmacology, but symptom control in and of itself is not taught.

The theme of symptom control as such evolved out of the hospice movement of about 30 years ago. As a result of research at St. Christopher's Hospice in London and later, the work of Robert Twycross (Twycross 1987), doctors have a pretty good idea how to manage most symptoms. Yet, there is no course in any medical school curriculum that looks at a classic cancer patient at the end of life, suffering a great deal from multiple symptoms (which include everything from pain to nausea, vomiting, hiccups, decubitus ulcers and more), as a single person having a range of symptoms. The medical staff doesn't look at that patient and evaluate the whole patient with all his or her symptoms. They don't go through the entire gamut of symptoms and find the appropriate treatment for each; that's not the way symptom control is solved today.

The specialist for any given symptom, whether a gastroenterologist, a neurologist, or someone else, is called in. Symptoms are handled in a piecemeal

33

fashion in most situations, as opposed to having a single physician involved in reviewing the total management of a given patient. That's an inherent problem in medical school education and, to a lesser degree, in nursing school education.

Changes have to be made in the way we teach some areas of medicine, and that's a huge job, as anyone who has tried to put changes through in a curriculum committee knows. No one tries to put through changes that would affect everything from the Department of Anatomy to the Departments of Physiology, Pharmacology, Internal Medicine and all the other sub-specialties. Dealing with departmental turf issues and changing relationships among faculty members is difficult. However, that is precisely what is called for in reviewing what doctors do and think about when they approach patient care.

No topic in patient care deserves as much attention as the topic of comfort. And it requires a change in thinking. In the next 20 years, we must completely reorient our approach to symptom control, both as a teaching modality and as a system which gathers together in a different way all the specialty disciplines that now do the job half-heartedly. It's not as though we have to reinvent the wheel. The knowledge is there; we have to coordinate it.

TRAINING IN ETHICS

A second major issue in the area of cancer education is the ethics of cancer treatment. Sporadic attempts have been made at Columbia and elsewhere to teach cancer ethics, but they have not been very successful and have never lasted for more than an experimental phase. There are many ethical issues faced by young students in training. Often they don't know they are facing such issues; when they do face them, they don't know to whom they should talk about them. They feel very troubled. They often watch their seniors bury these issues. They come away thinking that the way one approaches these issues is to bury them.

What are these ethical issues? They include everything from the manner of treatment available for different populations to the experimental protocols to which cancer patients are often subjected. Is continuation of care of a certain kind warranted for the sake of a patient or warranted for the sake of a protocol? At times, the issue of continuation of care has to do with how one addresses the end phase of life. At what point does one define a person as terminally ill to the extent that life support systems may seem almost obscene? These are ethical and moral issues—real dilemmas in medicine.

Some attempts have been made at Columbia-Presbyterian Medical Center to bring ethicists to the bedside to participate in some of the deliberating sessions. Such arrangements have been extremely stimulating, especially if the ethicist was a person who understood medicine.

Experts in religion, ethics, family therapy, and so on do exist in the outside world. The problem is, do those experts understand the world of medicine or are they really outsiders who have a body of knowledge, but who cannot understand the life of the physician who cares for the patient? What they have to offer sometimes fits and sometimes doesn't, in a haphazard way. For example, a well trained psychiatrist—an intelligent, sensitive, caring individual—comes onto a surgical unit and writes a recommendation in wonderful language, which nobody understands because it is purely the language of his or her specialty and, in fact, does not address the problem the surgeon faces, even though that is why that individual has been consulted. If psychiatrists don't find a way to make what they have to offer absolutely and practically relevant to those with whom they work or those who call upon them for their expertise, the wonderful things they may possibly have to say are absolutely useless. A language to communicate must be found that makes sense for a surgical unit.

It may be a very good thing to sit at the bedside and hold somebody's hand for two hours a day, but it is impossible for a surgeon in a busy surgical unit who hardly has five minutes to spare for each patient. To make such a recommendation, then, is silly and wasteful. The recommendation has to fit the resources of the unit.

If an ethicist comes to the bedside and does rounds with medical students, he or she may make a meaningful contribution. If, however, the same ethicist ends up with a very abstract, philosphical discussion about good and evil, nothing will be accomplished. The subject of ethics is important, but it has to apply to the bedside in a manner which is both economical in terms of time as well as dollars, and is meaningful and relevant for the students who are also at bedside.

The following story illustrates an ethical problem experienced by a budding psychiatrist when he was still undergoing the rotations of his internship. It was his turn to rotate through gynecology, which, at that time, was responsible for breast surgery as well. It was about 25 years ago, when the kind of surgery to be done was decided upon just when the breast biopsy was performed, and the patient would discover whether she had lost a breast or not only after the fact.

The young psychiatrist, in this case, was told to talk with the patient—a woman in her early thirties, about to be married. She was a professional woman who felt reasonably fulfilled in every aspect of her life except her personal life. The coming marriage was most important to her, especially since it represented her first sexual experience. Therefore, the potential mastectomy held enormous significance for her. Would she be left with a only a little scar or without a breast?

The surgeon left the emotional aspects of the case to the psychiatric student. He was prepared to handle the technical aspects. He reassured the woman that everything would be all right.

"How can you say that?" asked the psychiatrist. "You don't know. It doesn't feel benign." The surgeon responded, "Don't worry about it. That's the way the patients like it. You have to reassure them. I've had many years of experience."

None of the team knew what the outcome would be. When the woman woke up, she discovered that a radical mastectomy had been performed. How ethical were the reassurances offered her by the surgeon prior to the operation? The surgeon merely washed his hands of the case after he had completed the operation. It was left to others to handle the consequences.

The psychiatrist was the only one who knew what the woman was worried about with the respect to the implications a radical mastectomy would have on her impending marriage. He knew why she had to shriek in fury and dismay when she awoke in the recovery room.

The economics of medicine today is pushing all doctors into cutting that area of care out of the budget which is in fact the most relevant part of medicine; not the elegant stitches that leave no scar, but the emotional kind of stitching up which leaves the least amount of scar in terms of the person's feelings, sense of identity, sense of the future, and quality of life. That is ethics, and doctors have to find some way to bring that back into the vocabulary of medicine— every kind of medicine.

The burden of much that has been discarded from medical care has literally been dumped into the hands of social workers in this country. They are carrying it very well, given the resources they have, but the dumping is a medical issue that has ethical connotations: what responsibility has a medical practitioner to his or her patient? How far does that responsibility go? Where does it stop?

These are major issues. Can these things be taught? One way is by providing role models. Teachers may be role models in the way they relate to their patients and in what they worry about. Is theirs a nine-to-five job, for example? Or is it something beyond that? That's a role model issue. Another way of teaching responsibility is through discussion at the bedside.

TRAINING IN COMMUNICATION PATTERNS

The next topic that belongs in the cancer curriculum is a new specialty that we might call oncotherapy. Cancer therapy integrates disciplines of mental health into the field of cancer. An oncotherapist is someone from any discipline who specializes in the communication patterns specific to patients with cancer. It is an intriguing area. The way people talk and relate to one another when the diagnosis of cancer is made quickly reflects a difference in tone, in mood, and in language. People speak of having a tumor. What kind of tumor is it? It's a tumor that is growing faster than it should. Euphemisms are used to avoid the word cancer. It's an old issue. The word itself creates a vocabulary, a language, a communication pattern that interferes with clarity of statement, with clarity of stated options.

Fear of malpractice suits causes many physicians to have their patients sign informed consent forms that list every possible complication that may result from cancer treatments. Much of it is unnecessary. It scares many people. But we live in a litigious age. Because of the possibility of further complications, however, the notion of ongoing therapy is a valid one. One of the more complicated aspects of oncotherapy has to do with what happens in communication patterns within families. How, where, and from whom do families learn to talk about the illness? Clearly it is from those who surround the patient. The way the medical team behaves is very often the way families will behave. This may not always be to their benefit. A trained family therapist who understands the way families communicate and handle problems would be a most welcome addition to the medical team.

It is common for families to exclude children from certain conversations "for their own good." What happens in hospitals is similar. Even when the patient is an adult, the family steps outside the patient's room to talk to the doctor privately and the patient in bed just hears whispers but knows that they are talking about him. When the family returns and he asks what was discussed, evasive answers are given about the weather or Blue Cross or something else. These patterns of communication are used when people are anxious. Some of them may be very good, but some of them are not. A trained person would understand what was taking place and would be able to help direct and teach the family to handle matters in a better way. A family therapist is crucial in the field of cancer, probably more important than a psychiatrist, who is primarily trained in individual therapy techniques. They are important too, but a family therapist plays the key role.

How can training in communication patterns be handled in medical or nursing schools? Clearly, not everyone has to be an expert in every field,. In psychiatry, for example, residents in training must at least learn something about hyperthyroidism before they diagnose depression and start prescribing an antidepressant to a patient who may, in fact, have a low thyroid function. They must at least know something about the potential for brain dysfunction on an organic basis before they diagnose psychosis and give a phenothyazine to a patient in whom a tumor is growing. Regardless of specialty, doctors must be aware of the dimensions of treatment possibilities, and function, to some degree, as triage officers. The triage function has to be taught in medical school and will be very important in a cancer curriculum.

TRAINING IN STAFF SUPPORT

A final topic that belongs in a cancer curriculum—and it is often the most neglected area in cancer—is staff support. The image conjured up by the phrase "staff support" is that of supportive therapy. It may sound infantalizing, demeaning, or disrespectful to the individual. But everyone needs staff support when sinking in a sea of misery, when close to burnout, when overwhelmed. Support does not mean holding the person's hand. Staff support on a professional level means understanding how important it is to be aware of each other's warning signals, to be alert to a colleague's trouble. Trouble affects judgement and commitment to the patient. Doctors who are in trouble cannot focus their entire attention on their work. A doctor's inability to marshal his or her resources may negatively affect the patient's treatment.

Staff support means a disciplined, honest, professional, and sophisticated way of spotting trouble among colleagues. A system of weekly or monthly ward rounds in any given unit, during which physicians talk about what it's like to be doing what they are doing, and who is having a rough time or an easy time, is necessary. An outsider may be required to coordinate this. This is not group therapy, although it may have a flavor of it. It's a kind of recess, a time for letting one's hair down to review what works, what doesn't work, who needs to shift patients, what kinds of rotations are needed, and so on.

These kinds of issues are a very important dimension of cancer work. They are often neglected and should be built into every single unit which manages difficult patients.

REFERENCE

TWYCROSS, R. 1987. *Control of Alimentary Symptoms in Far Advanced Cancer.* New York: Churchill Livingstone Inc.

5

Factors Contributing to Poorly Relieved Pain in the Cancer Patient

Nessa Coyle, RN, MS

The fear of pain associated with cancer plays a major role in an individual's quality of life from time of diagnosis. This fear can be greater than the fear of death, and is perpetuated by stories of friends or relatives who experienced severe pain and suffering as their disease progressed. Clinical observations suggest that such fears may be well founded for many cancer patients. Prevalent surveys on the severity of pain indicate that moderate to severe pain is experienced by one third of patients in active therapy, and by 60–90 percent of patients with advanced disease (Twycross and Lack 1984). Although Foley (1979) suggests that pain in 90–95 percent of patients can be adequately controlled with current therapies, Twycross and Lack (1984) estimate that as many as 25 percent of cancer patients worldwide die without relief from severe pain (see also Daut and Cleeland 1982). A series of factors are implicated in why cancer pain is poorly managed. Usually these factors result in failure to believe the patient's pain level, or treatment focused too heavily on either psychological or physiological parameters. The patient and family may be labeled as being inadequate in some way, so that the blame for less than optimal pain relief is removed from the staff and placed instead on the family system.

ASSESSMENT FACTORS

Assessment is the first step in pain management; if incomplete, it will result in poorly controlled pain. Assessment of pain includes type of pain, whether acute or chronic; profile of the patient with pain; and categorization of the pain syndrome.

Type of Pain

Failure by health professionals to recognize the difference between acute and chronic pain is a source of poorly relieved pain in the chronic pain patient. The signs of acute pain parallel those of anxiety, with hyperactivity of the central nervous system. There is a well-defined pattern of onset, evidence of tissue damage, and resolution of pain with restoration of normal tissue function. For these patients, pain is usually well managed. However, in chronic pain—that is, pain persisting for a series of months or longer—the autonomic nervous system adapts, and the objective signs of acute pain are no longer present. The signs of chronic pain frequently parallel those of depression, and the patient's report of pain may be the only measure of its existence (Foley 1985). Chronic pain patients are at risk for having health professionals fail to believe the severity of their pain and identify their major problem as that of depression. Chronic pain does, however, lead to changes in personality, life style, and functional ability. Such pain requires an approach which deals not only with the cause of the pain, but also its psychological and social aftermath (Foley 1985).

Profile of Patients with Cancer Pain

Profiling patients with cancer pain is important. The meaning of the pain for that individual becomes clearer within the whole spectrum of the illness and the suffering component of the pain can be more clearly identified and addressed. Classification within five groups is helpful (Foley 1985; Coyle and Foley 1985).

> *Group one* includes patients with acute cancer-related pain. This pain may be a result of either the tumor or its treatment. If pain was the mark of the original cancer diagnosis, each new episode of pain is a reminder of that initial experience and the fear it evoked.
>
> *Group two* includes patients with chronic cancer-related pain. As with acute pain, chronic pain may be the result of tumor progression or of cancer treatment. With chronic pain associated with tumor progression, suffering plays a major role in the "total" pain experienced by patients.
>
> *Group three* includes patients with a history of chronic pain who develop cancer and pain. Frequently these patients and families are already psychologically exhausted; their coping resources have been stretched to the limit. Suffering can again be a major component in the pain experience.
>
> *Group four* includes patients with a history of drug addiction who have cancer-related pain. Within this grouping are patients who are actively using street drugs, patients who are in methadone maintenance programs, and patients who have not used drugs for many years. These patients are

most vunerable to having their pain poorly managed. The first subgroup can strain the resources of even the most sophisticated pain management team. The second and third subgroups do not present a management problem. However, recognition is required that these patients are at risk for recidivism because of the high stress associated with cancer and pain. It must also be recognized that these patients are tolerant to narcotics because of previous drug use. A higher dosage of drug than is normally anticipated may be required to control their pain.

Group five includes patients who are dying of cancer and are in pain. At no time is poorly controlled pain more destructive, not only to the patient, but also to family and staff. For these patients, the psychological consequences of pain compound those of death and dying.

Categorization of Pain Syndromes

Pain syndromes occuring in patients with cancer may be general or specific. General syndromes include those associated with any debilitating disease. They may include cumulative physical and social losses, and frequently encompass much suffering. Specific pain syndromes lie within three major areas: pain associated with direct tumor involvement, pain associated with cancer therapy, and pain unrelated to cancer or its treatment (Coyle and Foley 1985). Inadequate assessment of the changing nature of pain, and the multiple sources of pain and suffering in the advanced cancer patient, lead to inadequate pain relief.

COMMUNICATION FACTORS

A communication gap between the patient and health professionals is not uncommon and can be another source of increased suffering for the patient with pain. The risk of poor communication is heightened by the subjective nature of pain, and by the combination of physiological and psychological factors in the pain experience. Paying attention to the words used by the patient to describe the pain is helpful in determining its etiology and alerts one to the suffering component. Medical and nursing staff can enhance communication both directly, by believing without reserve that the intensity of the pain is at the level reported by the patient, and indirectly, by observing levels of activity prior to and following pain relief measures. Some patients benefit by communicating their pain through means of a body chart, coloring in each site of pain and marking its severity.

This involvement enhances a patient's sense of participation and control. Current research on the development of a valid instrument for the assessment of pain in the patient with cancer addresses both the pain and the suffering components (Fishman et al 1985). Each needs to be addressed if the pain is to be adequately managed. If this tool is validated, it will be an extremely useful method for the patient to describe his or her experience in a way understood by the physician and nurse.

Because of the multidisciplinary nature of pain management, poor communication among team members can result in fragmentation of care. This is minimized when one team member, usually a nurse clinician, assumes the primary-liaison coordinating role between team and patient (Coyle et al. 1985).

FACTORS SURROUNDING THE USE OF NARCOTICS

Many factors contribute to the inadequate use of narcotic analgesics. These include fear of respiratory depression; lack of understanding of the difference between tolerance, physical dependence, and psychological dependence; fear of psychological dependence (addiction); and lack of knowledge of equianalgesic doses of drugs related to route of administration. This fear and lack of knowledge frequently results in undue concern with the milligram dose of a drug, rather than using the patient's response to the drug as the indicator of whether the dose being administered is sufficient. Unlike nonsteroidal anti-inflammatory drugs, there is no ceiling effect with narcotic analgesic (Foley 1982). This implies that there is no absolute milligram dose of the drug beyond which one cannot go. The limiting factor is unacceptable side effects experienced by the patient. Those seen most frequently in the tolerant patient are confusion, hallucinations, and sedation (Catalano 1985).

Tolerance is described as the requirement of increasing amounts of the narcotic to achieve adequate pain relief (Foley 1985). It is most frequently seen in patients with advancing disease. The phenomenon of tolerance is not clearly understood, but is felt to occur at a receptor level (Inturrisi and Foley 1984). Routes of administration affect the rapidity with which tolerance develops. The epidural and intrathecal route is the most rapid, followed by the intravenous route. Next comes the intramuscular or subcutaneous route, and finally the oral route (Foley 1982). Oral administration is the preferred route not only because of the tolerance factor, but because it is least invasive for the patient and more easy to manage by the family in the home setting. With narcotics, cross tolerance is not complete. This means that patients receiving high doses of narcotics to control their pain who experience adverse side effects can be switched to a different narcotic at an equianalgesic starting dose of approximately 50 percent. The dose is then titrated up or down depending on the patient's response (Foley 1982).

The fear of respiratory depression is a major reason for underprescribing narcotic analgesics for cancer-related pain, and yet narcotic-induced respiratory depression is uncommon in the tolerant patient. These patients rapidly develop tolerance to the respiratory depressant effects of the drugs (Catalano 1985).

Physical dependence is an expected outcome in patients who use narcotic analgesics on a regular basis for a period of approximately two weeks or longer. The patient may show signs of withdrawal if the drug is stopped abruptly, but will not have a psychological craving for the drug (Porter and Hick 1980). The patient is not psychologically dependent (addicted), but may label him or herself as such, or be labelled by others in this way, unless the phenomenon is understood by patient, family, and staff alike. This understanding is particularly important in the advanced cancer patient who undergoes a neuroablative procedure, experiences relief of pain, and no longer requires narcotic analgesics. If the narcotic is stopped abruptly, the patient may exhibit signs and symptoms of withdrawal and equate this with addiction. Withdrawal signs and symptoms can be prevented by administering 25 percent of the previous twenty-four-hour narcotic requirements and slowly diminishing the dose over several days (Foley 1982), the pace being determined by the patient's response.

On very rare occasions, the cancer patient on an around-the-clock regimen of narcotics to control pain is given naloxone, a narcotic antagonist, to establish whether a sudden change in level of alertness is the result of narcotic accumulation. It is important to remember that if this antagonist is given in a bolus of 0.4 mg intravenously, the patient will be put into withdrawal and will experience in that instance all the pain that has been supressed by the narcotic. The patient may become psychotic from this abrupt flooding of consciousness with severe pain. In the rare instance that naloxone is indicated for a patient in this group, the drug should be diluted in 10cc of normal saline and slowly titrated to the patient's respirations (Foley 1982). In this way the sudden flooding of consciousness by pain is prevented. The tolerant patient is more sensitive to the antagonist group of drugs than the nontolerant patient, and is therefore put more easily into withdrawal.

Psychological dependence (addiction) contains elements of physical dependence and tolerance but is unique in that there is an overriding craving for the drug whether pain is present or not. Although psychological dependence occurs in under 1 percent of patients using narcotics for cancer-related pain (Porter and Hick 1980), societal fear of such drugs is profound. The mood-altering effects, unrelated to pain, sought after by street addicts color the way narcotics are prescribed and administered to relieve pain. This uneasiness toward prescribing and administering escalating doses of narcotics, even for the advanced cancer patient, arises from the recognition that pain is subjective, that gauging severity of pain is based on the patient's word, and that prescribing and administering the drug is based on belief in the patient's word. In clinical experience, if the staff has a sense that the patient is using the narcotic to "feel good'' as well as to relieve pain, the administration of the drug may then become a moral issue in the eyes of the staff or family, and the drug may be withheld, given in smaller amounts, or given at greater intervals than is required to prevent pain breakthrough.

Lack of knowledge of equianalgesic doses of drugs depending on the route of administration can also reinforce this fear of psychological dependence (addiction). Because of the "first pass" effect, narcotics, when taken by the oral route, may need to be taken in amounts from two to five times that of the parenteral route (Catalano 1985). Although this information is readily available in the pain literature, deep-seated fear of narcotics sometimes overrides the rational prescription and administration of these drugs.

REFERENCES

CATALANO, R. 1985. "Pharmacology of Analgesics." *Seminars in Oncology Nursing* 1(2):126–139.

COYLE, N. AND K. FOLEY. 1985. "Pain in Patients with Cancer: Profile of Patients and Common Pain Syndromes." *Seminars in Oncology Nursing* 1(2):93–99.

COYLE, N., E. MONZILLO, M. LOSCALZO, C. FARKAS, M. J. MASSIE, AND K. M. FOLEY. 1985. "A Model of Continuity of Care for Cancer Patients with Pain and Neuro-oncologic Complications." *Cancer Nursing* 8:111–119.

DAUT, R. L. AND C. S. CLEELAND. 1982. "The Prevalance and Severity of Pain in Cancer." *Cancer* 50:1932–1938.

FISHMAN, B., S. PASTERNAK, S. WALLENSTEIN, R. W. HOUDE, J. HOLLAND, AND K. M. FOLEY. 1985. "The Memorial Pain Assessment Card." Presented at the annual meeting of the American Pain Society, October, Dallas, Texas.

FOLEY, K. M. 1979. "The Management of Pain of Malignant Origin." In H. R. Tyler and D. M. Dawson, eds. *Current Neurology.* New York: Houghton Mifflin, pp. 279–302.

FOLEY, K. M. 1982. "The Practical Use of Narcotic Analgesics." In M. M. Reidenberg, ed. *The Medical Clinics of North America.* Philadelphia: W. B. Saunders, pp. 1091–1104.

FOLEY, K. 1985. "The Treatment of Cancer Pain." *New England Journal of Medicine* 313:84–95.

INTURRISI, C. E. AND K. M. FOLEY. 1984. "Narcotic Analgesics in the Management of Pain." In M. Kuhar and G. Pasternak, eds. *Analgesics: Neurochemical, Behavioral and Clinical Perspectives.* New York: Raven Press, pp. 257–287.

TWYCROSS, R. G. AND S. LACK. 1984. *Symptom Control in Far Advanced Cancer: Pain Relief.* London: Pitman.

PORTER, J. AND H. HICK. 1980. " Addicition Rare in Patients Treated with Narcotics." *New England Journal of Medicine* 302:123.

6

Psychosocial Interventions with Cancer Patients and Their Families

Francine Cournos, MD

Mr. Smith was 80 years old when he first tried to take his life. He was hospitalized for prostate cancer, which had metastasized widely to his bones, and he was in a great deal of pain.

The medical staff understood Mr. Smith's motivation to take his life. At least they thought they did. He had only months to live. He was in great pain, both from his disease and from the treatment for it. It was, from the staff's point of view, a perfectly rational choice to decide to suffer no longer. But since it was hospital policy that a psychiatrist be called in after all suicide attempts, a consultant came in to ask Mr. Smith the obvious question: why had he cut his wrists with a razor blade the previous night? The answer turned out to be less obvious than the question.

Mr. Smith explained that his sister had died a week ago, and that he had learned this only the night before from a distant acquaintance who had called to offer condolences. Mr. Smith's family had withheld the news, thinking they would spare him unnecessary pain. But that was not Mr. Smith's interpretation of their behavior. He felt that if his family would no longer share important news with him, they must have already written him off as dead, so he might as well not exist.

The psychiatrist spoke with the family, bringing them together to achieve some better understanding of what had happened. The family reassured Mr. Smith that he was still important. Mr. Smith apologized, expressing a strong desire to go on living now that he knew he was still a part of the family. He was pleased to go home, where he spent the four months left to him without any further self-destructive acts. The staff, for their part, were humbled to learn that it was not pain or terminal cancer that had made Mr. Smith feel such despair, but the worry that his cancer had excluded him from his family.

Mr. Smith's case demonstrates that the emotional needs of cancer patients and their families are far from self-evident. The following themes are common.

HELPING PATIENTS MAINTAIN CONTROL

Hospital staff are experts, and often they want to impose their expertise by telling patients and families what is best. But people don't want simply to follow advice. They want a say in what is going to happen.

Mrs. Lipton, a 52-year-old woman with metastatic colon cancer, terminated treatment with an oncologist who showed contempt for her plans to switch to a macrobiotic diet. The new oncologist approved of this step, and even suggested some books on the subject. Mrs. Lipton felt understood and was fully cooperative with the traditional chemotherapy regimen that the new doctor recommended. Mr. and Mrs. Lipton knew other cancer victims who had great faith in this diet. The diet became their way of fighting the cancer, and they needed to have their own efforts affirmed.

HELPING PATIENTS DISCUSS THEIR CONCERNS

Many patients with cancer do not discuss their worries because they fear this would burden others. Often families misinterpret this reserve as the patient's fear of accepting and discussing the illness. As with Mr. Smith, the family may be trying to protect the patient by avoiding painful subjects, but the result is that the patient feels isolated. Hospital staff can help bridge that gap. By hearing out the patient and his family, staff can understand the needs of each and help create better communication.

More than half the patients admitted to one cancer ward of a general hospital had never discussed the diagnosis of cancer with family members. Families would tell staff the patient didn't know what was wrong, and patients would tell staff that they themselves were concealing their knowledge of the disease from their families. Often in this situation, patients feel progressively more isolated and frightened to confide in anyone. While not every patient wants to hear about the diagnosis of cancer, the overwhelming majority eventually figure it out. They have questions about the illness and its treatment and need to settle their affairs if they are near death.

Sometimes staff are as reluctant as families to hear about patients' concerns. Mrs. Cooper was a 45-year-old woman with lung cancer metastatic to bone. Her attending physician refused to tell her what was wrong. She kept requesting more information from other staff, but they had been prohibited from offering any by her physician. One day, the medical resident got up the courage to respond to Mrs. Cooper's inquiry by asking her how she herself understood the problem. Mrs. Cooper replied by saying that she assumed she had cancer, that it had spread, and that she would not live much longer. The resident told her that she had succeeded in figuring out her own situation quite accurately. Mrs. Cooper then said that it was helpful to know for sure, because she was divorced, and needed to make plans for her 15-year-old son. Thereafter, Mrs. Cooper was able to concentrate on her physical comfort rather than pressing the staff for her diagnosis. She became calmer and was more willing to request necessary pain medication. In spite of these improvements in Mrs. Cooper, the attending physician was enraged that the patient now knew her diagnosis. This is a startling example of the way information ostensibly withheld to protect a patient is actually being withheld to shield the staff or family.

HELPING PATIENTS MAINTAIN HOPE

Cancer patients and their families, no matter how educated and rational they are, maintain magical hopes of a cure. These hopes, while serving a necessary and valuable purpose, often require a response from the staff. Sensitive staff quickly discern what patients are ready to hear and what they need to avoid hearing. One mother expressed concern that the chemotherapy her 20-year-old daughter was receiving for lymphoma might cause another cancer later on. While this was a real concern, she was also expressing the hope that her daughter had a long-term future and minimizing the present threat of her disease.

Confronting an unrealistic belief may sometimes be necessary. Mr. Edwards was a 60-year-old man whose 58-year-old wife was in the terminal phase of metastatic ovarian cancer. The couple had been married for 26 years. There were no children, and they had grown extremely dependent on one another. Mr. Edwards spent all his days at the hospital. He was terrified of his wife's impending death, and even refused to believe that it would occur. Mr. Edwards listened angrily to staff reports about his wife's deteriorating condition, and held to his position. He also refused psychiatric help. Mr. Edwards was present at the moment of his wife's death. He threw himself on his wife's body, kissing her repeatedly and refusing to allow her to be taken to the hospital morgue. When, eventually, staff insisted that the body be removed, Mr. Edwards ran from the hospital without another word to anyone. His reaction provides a vivid example of how far denial can go.

On the other hand, patients and families feel it is cruel to be confronted unnecessarily with the fatal nature of the illness. One patient was told, "You're a walking time-bomb," another that her treatment "was only palliative" and would have no influence on her lifespan. Sensitive staff control what they say to convey the facts without unnecessarily destroying the patient's hope.

CONCLUSION

Sensitivity to the psychosocial aspects of cancer management will help patients and families maintain hope, control, and social contact. Front-line staff are in the best position to understand and respond to the problems that arise in a particular situation. Listening to what patients and families say is an essential first step. Carefully weighing the balance between conveying accurate information and providing protection from overwhelmingly negative information will then follow. Helping patients and families maintain emotional closeness with one another is also crucial. Even where death is imminent and inevitable, these measures continue to provide comfort and support.

7

Clinical Cancer Education
in the Pediatric Setting

Anneliese Sitarz, MD

As recently as 30 years ago, the diagnosis of cancer was almost inevitably a death sentence, and the treatment of a patient with cancer was limited to surgery, radiotherapy, and emotional support. Since that time, much has been learned about differences in various types of cancer, prognostic factors that may be useful in determining the extent or type of treatment needed, and the importance of evaluating the extent of disease in a given patient. Also, the discovery of numerous chemicals that have shown effectiveness against various forms of cancer has given the medical staff a much broader treatment armamentarium.

Despite these facts and the curability of many forms of cancer, many patients still die of the disease, or of the consequences of the disease or its treatment. The medical staff has an increasingly complex task to learn about the intricacies of the various forms of cancer, the therapeutic measures for each type or stage of cancer, and also the potential short- or long-term consequences of these therapies. The latter has particular significance for pediatric patients. Children not only must survive the disease, but continue to grow and mature.

The pediatric oncologist must therefore be especially careful in delineating the extent and stage of disease in order to tailor the treatment to the given patient and limit unnecessary side effects. Delineating the extent of disease necessarily involves various surgical and radiological measures, and these too must be used with care to avoid damage to the growing patient or to that patient's quality of life. There is a relatively narrow margin between curing the cancer and not interfering with the child's normal development—and this is true in both medical and psychological terms.

Dealing with cancer in pediatric patients is particularly demanding for the medical staff. These days, most physicians who take care of children expect their patients to do well. Having to make a diagnosis of cancer in a child, and thus having to face the possible maiming or death of that child, is of course emotionally difficult. The physician must learn to deal with his or her own emotions before being able to help the patients or their families.

While the infant or young toddler will not ask questions, the older child will. It can be very difficult to remain honest and still not destroy that child's hope and trust. The parents and relatives need help with this, too. Thus the physician caring for a child with cancer must in fact deal with the whole family and becomes the "family physician."

One of the first and greatest tasks for the medical staff who are treating cancer patients is to try to understand where the parents and the older children are in their perception of what is going on. This assessment involves the parents' educational level, ethnic background, social status, emotional stability, and coping mechanisms. It also should include awareness of the psychodynamics within the family as well as of the extended family. Who is there who could lend support to (or occasionally interfere with) the family's coping? How are the parents dealing with the inevitable feelings of guilt regarding the child's illness?

Since many childhood cancers grow extremely rapidly, expediency of evaluating the patient is important. This need creates a stressful situation for the physician, the parents and the patient. The physician must try to explain as much as possible about the disease to the family at a time when they are reeling from shock at having been told the diagnosis. The parents, having heard the diagnosis, want treatment as quickly as possible and may find it hard to accept some of the inevitable delays that come with scheduling radiologic evaluations or operating room time. The need for careful and extensive evaluation to localize tumor and allow careful tailoring of treatment may not be appreciated at first when, having heard the word "cancer," the parents have difficulty hearing anything else and push to get treatment started. In addition, the child, especially a younger one, will find the procedures frightening and the perceived anxiety of the parents additionally unnerving. Even a young child's fears must be dealt with and simple explanations given for what is being done.

What the child is told needs to be commensurate with his or her ability to understand, and is thus age-dependent. From about three years of age on, the child will usually cooperate much more readily if he or she is given some explanation of what is going on. Time taken to do this is a worthwhile investment in establishing a good relationship with that child. Even at this age, the patients understand a lot more than one would think possible, if an appropriate effort is made to help them do so; they need not only explanations of any procedures being done, but also some concept of the chronicity of the disease—that it is not just a cold!

Once the diagnosis is made, the treatment plan must be outlined to the parents and the older patient. This may involve randomization to one of several regimens on protocols. Parents are often frightened by this prospect, and question the "guinea pig" aspect of it. The physician is often asked what he or she would do in the parents' place. Parents may have difficulty in understanding the rationale behind randomized treatment regimens, and this rationale must be explained to them. In many cases the randomization is in terms of intensity or duration of treatment; in others it may either include or exclude a modality such as radiotherapy. Usually the reason relates to maximizing treatment and minimizing side effects. It is important for the physician to have enough background information, such as results of previous treatments, to explain this, and to do so in terms the parents and older patient can understand. The risks and benefits must be put in proper perspective. Assurance must also be given that treatment will be stopped or changed if the desired results are not achieved or if serious side effects are experienced. Potential adverse reactions must be outlined, but this should clearly be done in such a way that the parents are not left with the feeling that the treatment is worse than the disease. Having a social worker or pediatric psychiatric nurse also meet with the parents to discuss these issues is important in helping parents reach a decision regarding treatment. Parents feel less helpless if they know that they are part of the treatment *team*. They know their child best and can best interpret his or her reactions to the medical staff. In general, the more the parents (and the patient) understand what is being done, the better their compliance. Also, the better the understanding, the more likely that the interaction of the family with the medical staff will be positive.

The diagnosis of cancer is not only frightening, it leads to anger. "Why did this happen to me (or my child)?" This anger is commonly directed at the staff and may be overt or indirect. For example, the child may show his anger by refusing to take medication—especially if he or she feels well and the medication leads to nausea. The physician is then confronted with the dilemma of having to convince the child of the need for continuing medication without frightening him unnecessarily about the disease. The parents are torn between their own fear of the drugs and the knowledge that these drugs are crucial to the child's survival. In other instances, parents may show anger by endless complaints about relatively insignificant things. Health professionals must be able to deal with this anger without responding in kind. It is important, first of all, not to take the anger personally. In order to help the family, staff must learn to remain objective about the anger, try to get the family to understand *why* they are angry, and help them deal with it. This can be very frustrating, difficult and exhausting. If the child is not doing well, the frustration is accentuated.

Nonetheless, the professional must learn to deal with this frustration—without taking it home!

Often, parents can be helped by involving them as much as possible in the child's care and by stressing that they are important members of the treatment team. For some parents this involvement is limited to the physical care of the child. For others it includes getting information about alternative treatments or new drugs. This should be condoned to the extent that the information they get is discussed and evaluated in an objective way. One can encourage them to read or bring in medical articles if they find something that interests them. This may reduce the tendency to "shop" for different treatments. It also reduces the feeling of helplessness that is probably the most terrible feeling parents have to endure. The less helpless the parents can be made to feel, the better they will be able to cope with their own emotions and to support the child.

Parents vary in their desire to be with the child during procedures such as bone marrow aspirations or spinal taps, and their wishes in this regard should be respected. In general, the child is less frightened if the parents remain with him or her. If, however, the parent does not feel comfortable remaining in the room, this should not be forced. A young physician may also feel insecure performing the procedure with the parents looking on. This too should be understood. Often, however, the parents can be encouraged to keep their eyes on the child and thus not on the procedure—if this helps the physician. For many, if not most parents, being in the room—even during an unpleasant procedure—is easier than standing outside and hearing the child scream. Being present can also help the parents understand what is happening and thus support the child better in dealing with it; for most parents, the known or observed is less frightening than the unknown. Their presence also supports their understanding that they are part of the team.

For many parents the extended family lends much support; this should be encouraged by including them in meetings with the staff so that as much information as possible is disseminated to them. Information given to the other family members, such as grandparents, aunts, and uncles, not only helps them to understand the situation, but also reduces the likelihood that these well-meaning people will try to undermine the treatment by questioning the diagnosis or suggesting inappropriate treatment measures such as megavitamins or quack drugs.

Family members can help by dividing visiting hours with the parents, by finding blood donors, by arranging transportation, and so on. Here, too, involvement allays frustration and lends support to the parents and the child. Some parents refuse to leave the child's bedside, even for meals, and relatives can sometimes help by taking turns with them. In other instances where parents must go to work to hold their jobs, members of the extended family can be with the child during some of that time, thus making the parents feel more at ease about being away from the hospital.

Just as presenting the initial diagnosis and planned treatment to the parents and to the patient is a demanding time for the medical staff, so it is when a decision must be made about the possibility of stopping treatment. When the patient is doing well, the anxiety about stopping is balanced by the wish to reduce the risks associated with the potential side effects of chemotherapy. The older patient and the family should be given a clear understanding of the pros and cons in order to be able to accept the decision regarding the length of, or need for, treatment. Although initially, at diagnosis, the thought of potentially damaging chemotherapy is frightening for most families, it later serves a supportive function. Therefore stopping it is, for many families, secondary only to diagnosis in its traumatic impact. The more the parents have been allowed to participate in decision making, and the more they understand about the drugs, the easier it is for them to accept a decision to stop.

Much more difficult is the need to determine whether to stop treatment when the patient is doing poorly and is obviously not responding to the chemotherapy. This is especially true if the patient fails to respond or relapses after having responded to treatment earlier. The family's hopes are dashed, and the stress experienced by the physicians and nurses who have cared for that patient increases and may become intense. Frustration and anger may surface. This adds to the difficulty of dealing with the situation and must be recognized. The feelings, anxieties, questions and needs of the family must be taken into account when a decision to stop chemotherapy is being considered, but the parents should not have the burden of making that decision alone. Since they inevitably feel guilty about their child's illness already, this guilt should not potentially be exacerbated by having the parents decide when to stop treatment. They should clearly be a part of that decision making, however, along with the physician—again, as members of the team.

The child—especially the older child—must also be considered and his or her fears, anxieties, wishes taken into account. One may not wish to ask the child directly about stopping treatment, but one can often sense from what the child says what his or her feelings are in this regard.

Physicians and nurses have to be able and willing to recognize the point at which continuing aggressive therapy is unlikely to bring positive results and, in fact, will only prolong the patient's pain. They must also be able and willing to gently express their concern about this reality to the family. They must make it clear that stopping such treatments as chemotherapy does not mean stopping supportive care, and stress that all efforts to make the child comfortable will be continued.

When a patient is terminal or has died, the most trying lesson an oncologist must learn is to be able to feel for and with the patient and the family but not be so involved that a certain degree of objectively is not retained. While there is certainly no harm in feeling or sharing sadness, the physician's and nurses must remember that the family looks to them for guidance and support. A degree of objectivity is thus absolutely necessary. This is often difficult if the relationship with the family has been a long one.

It is not always easy for health professionals to leave the problems at the hospital, but each person must learn some way to do this if he or she is to survive in this area of practice and continue to help patients optimally through these trying times. For some the answer lies in hobbies or outside interests; for others the best solution is to remain at a distance, having as little personal involvment as possible. Some people cannot cope emotionally and should not be dealing with these patients at all. This coping mechanism almost always has to be learned. Some younger physicians cope by becoming "task oriented." Others tend to avoid caring for cancer patients. It is definitely easier for the physician to remain a bit more detached than for nurses; the doctor sees the patient only at intervals, while the nurses may care for the patient eight to twelve hours a day!

The age of the patient also influences this relationship. Younger staff members may tend to identify with the older adolescent and thus make an objective stance much more difficult. Some older staff members may tend to identify more with the parents than with the child and have more difficulty in remaining objective with the parents.

The current trend toward managing oncology patients by rotating staff coverage is partly an attempt to lessen the stress of caring for these patients. On the negative side of this, however, the patient is less likely to develop a close physician–patient relationship, which is extremely important in a chronic illness.

For many patients who appear to be cured of their childhood cancer and want to lead normal adult lives, there are continuing problems. Physicians need to be aware of this. Despite the fact that these patients are long-term survivors and appear well, their history of having had cancer may be an impediment in their choice of career. They may not get accepted by the military; they may have trouble getting insurance; they may be fearful of getting married, of getting pregnant, or of having abnormal children. Also, increasingly, we are seeing secondary cancers in some of the long-term survivors. One cannot be sure if the latter are related to the treatment the child received or to the fact that the patient had cancer in the first place and may be genetically "cancer prone." At any rate, long-term follow-up and support are necessary—even of those patients who seem to be well. This can be difficult because, as the children get older, they reject medical follow-up if they seem to be well, and in our mobile society they may be lost to follow-up because they have moved to another state. Yet such follow-up is extremely important, not only for the welfare of these individual patients but also to contribute to the statistical knowledge base.

We need to determine what the long-term outcome is for those people who are the first large cohort of childhood cancer survivors. These data could be helpful in reducing the stigma that currently keeps them from certain careers and in counselling them more specifically in terms of marriage and parenting.

All childhood cancer patients should be referred to major cancer centers for diagnosis and treatment. This serves several purposes. First, as stated previously, specific "front-end" investigations are providing new information that is important in tailoring treatment as much as possible to the exact stage and specific need of each form of cancer. In this way, the risk of untoward late effects of treatment in long-term survivors may be reduced. Second, information is gathered about the histologic characteristics and subclasses of various cancers that is increasingly important in tailoring the extent of therapy. Since most of these cancers are rare, only large centers would be likely to see enough of any one of them to collect such data. Third, cancer registries in such cancer centers not only quantify patient numbers, but may enhance the ability to get long-term follow-up. This would help us to answer some of the outstanding questions concerning the quality of life of the survivors.

8

The Cancer Educator as Role Model:
A Means of Initiating Attitude Change

Salvatore J. Bertolone, MD
Pamela Scott, RN, BSN

Over the past few decades, cancer education has received increasing attention from both the clinical and research points of view. As physicians have moved toward a more interventionist posture, there is increased use of early screening techniques, application of adjuvant chemotherapy and the acceptance of clinical research trials. For the patient with cancer, the physician–patient relationship assumes particular importance. Yet, according to a study by Krant (1976), 98 percent of cancer patients reported that their technical care was excellent but 60 percent stated their "needs" were not met by the physician. In response, cancer educators have recently begun to look at how students and others can be sensitized to the psychosocial needs of the cancer patient and how those needs can be met. There is now a greater emphasis on nonverbal communication in the doctor–patient relationship. Physician behavior, caring, and openness cannot be inferred from paper and pencil measures: They must be transmitted directly.

Three major issues affecting the attitudes of health professionals towards cancer and cancer patients can be identified. First, students and staff commonly maintain negative attitudes toward cancer and the cancer patient, owing in part to the belief that the cancer patient is a dying patient (Cohen et al. 1982). Second, according to the research of Haley and colleagues with the Cancer Attitude Survey (1977), medical students and house staff underestimate the cancer patient's ability to cope with diagnostic and prognostic information. The third issue may be the most significant of all and may be responsible, directly or indirectly, for the other two issues. Students and staff, in an effort to cope with the anxiety associated with their own personal developmental issues, tend to focus solely on the biological/technical aspects of medicine, thereby isolating themselves from the psychological and social issues confronting themselves, the cancer patient, and the patient's family (Frankel and Rosenblum 1983). These are the major issues facing cancer educators who are favorably disposed to promoting the biopsychosocial or holistic approach to medicine. In this chapter we will examine how the University of Louisville's Pediatric Hematology/ Oncology section is endeavoring to overcome these barriers.

Each member of the pediatric oncology section functions as a cancer educator and role model. Such role modeling is proving to be a powerful means of influencing student and staff attitudes. Experience has shown us that our attitudes as role models are best transmitted to students and house officers by informal methods (Blanchard et al. 1983). This is not to devalue formal, didactic cancer education, but rather to highlight the role of informal interactional clinical cancer education, particularly in exploring the psychosocial aspects of cancer.

Children with cancer, on and off therapy, are most frequently seen in the outpatient pediatric oncology clinic. In this setting, students from varying health care professions such as medicine, nursing, and art therapy often have their first contact with the pediatric cancer patient. The clinic setting has demonstrated its usefulness in cancer education, particularly in negating the belief that all cancer patients are dying. The majority of children being seen take an active part in life as manifested through their school attendance, play, and personal interactions. Since more than 70 percent of children diagnosed with cancer can be cured (Hammond 1985), students are being exposed to greater numbers of "cured" children. Also, according to a study done by Hays and colleagues (1985), it is in the outpatient setting, through their interactions with the children, that students begin to perceive the child as having inner emotional resources that permit adjustment to the problems presented by cancer and cancer therapy. Our experience with students supports this. Owing to the positive influence of the outpatient setting on student attitudes regarding cancer, the University of Louisville's pediatric residency program now requires one-month mandatory rotations for the pediatric residents through the out-patient clinic.

It is frequently reiterated that children and families have the ability to cope with the diagnostic information given to them about cancer (Cohen et al. 1982). The diagnosis and treatment of cancer is openly discussed with all patients, regardless of age, in terms that they can understand. The expectation is that the child and family will become active members of the health care team. In turn, students and staff are also expected to act as "team players." Inherent in being a team member is that information and support are mutually provided. Open sharing of information between child, family, and staff is vital, and questioning is encouraged. Students and staff who are truly comfortable in the team member role are encouraged to explore and identify what information needs to be shared with those families who have no specific questions. Becoming a "team player" takes practice and students and staff need help in learning that saying, "I don't know" is acceptable, and that it is imperative to look for guidance and support from other team members. What better way for young students or struggling house officers to address their own defensiveness and insecurity, than to have the chief of the oncology service tell the patient and family, "This is a team effort and no one person always has all the answers," and on occasion to admit, "I don't know the answer to that specific question, but I'll check it out for you."

Primary to the health team concept is the biopsychosocial approach to patient care. With guidance, students and staff can identify and address psychosocial patient/family concerns. Often they project their own personal feelings about a situation and then label those feelings as patient/family concerns. They must be assisted in differentiating where these feelings and issues originate—within themselves or within the patient/family unit. Students and staff often identify feelings of inadequacy when dealing with psychosocial issues once they are identified.

To illustrate: a thirteen-year-old diagnosed with osteogenic sarcoma who had been on chemotherapy for approximately six weeks presented to our institution for an above-the-knee amputation. During the previous six weeks the family had been assisted in openly discussing the operation, and they had the opportunity to meet another teenage patient with osteogenic sarcoma who had an amputated limb. The patient and family expressed that they had become as comfortable as possible with their decision for surgery. Upon admission, the students and staff manifested anxiety about the impending amputation of this teenager's leg and they recommended psychiatric intervention to provide emotional support for the family. When instructed to question the patient and family about how they felt they were coping, the staff responded that the patient and family felt they were coping well. With encouragement, the students and staff were able to openly express the anxiety they personally felt about this teenager's amputation. They also expressed fear that the family or patient would ask them questions to which they had no answers. It was related that families and patients do not expect answers to "ultimate" questions, rather they desire a supportive and attentive listener. Once the students' and staff's anxieties were acknowledged and dealt with openly, they were then able to move into a supportive role that proved beneficial to both staff and family.

It appears that during the clinical years of medical school, messages regarding cancer and its treatment become more complex. Cancer educators must compete as role models. It has been suggested that medical students tend to adopt attitudes paralleling those of their role models (Blanchard 1981). Through role modeling, several things can be accomplished. First, exposing students and house staff to interactions in the pediatric oncology clinic setting can help to dispel the belief that the cancer patient is necessarily a dying patient. Secondly, students and staff who are directed in open, supportive communication with patients and families, can become more aware that patients and families *can* cope with the diagnosis of cancer. Finally, by using the team approach, students and staff are better able to legitimize their feelings and reactions associated with personal developmental issues, and also to effectively address patient/family psychosocial concerns.

REFERENCES

BLANCHARD, C. G., J. C. RUCKDESCHEL, E. B. BLANCHARD, J. G. ARENA, N. L. SAUNDERS, AND E. D. MALLOY. 1983. "Interactions between Oncologists and Patients During Rounds." *Annals of Internal Medicine* 99:694–699.

BLANCHARD, C. G., M. D. RUCKDESCHEL, R. E. COHEN, E. S. SHAW, J. MCSHARRY, AND J. HORTON. 1981. "Attitudes Toward Cancer I: The Impact of a Comprehensive Oncology Course on Second-Year Medical Students." *Cancer* 47:2756–2762.

COHEN, R. E., J. C. RUCKDESCHEL, C. G. BLANCHARD, M. ROHRBAUGH, AND J. HORTON. 1982. "Attitudes Toward Cancer II: A Comparative Analysis of Cancer Patients, Medical Students, Medical Residents, Physicians and Cancer Educators." *Cancer* 50:1218–1223.

FRANKEL, B. L. AND S. ROSENBLUM. 1983. "Teaching a Biopsychosocial Approach on Medical Attending Rounds." *General Hospital Psychiatry* 5:133–140.

HALEY, H. B., H. HUYNH, R. E. A. PAIVA, AND I. R. JAUN. 1977. "Student Attitudes Toward Cancer: Changes in Medical School." *Journal of Medical Education* 52:500–507.

HAMMOND, G. D. 1985. "Multidisciplinary Clinical Investigation of the Cancers of Children: A Model for the Management of Adults with Cancer." *Cancer* 55(6):1215–1225.

HAYS, D. M., K. I. HOFFMAN, K. O. WILLIAMS, S. E. SIEGEL, AND R. MILLER. 1985. "Medical Students' Concepts of Childhood Cancer and its Management." *Medical and Pediatric Oncology* 13:78–82.

KRANT, M J. 1976. "Problems of the Physician in Presenting the Patient with the Diagnosis." In J. W. Cullen, B. H. Fox, and R. N. Osom, eds. *Cancer: The Behavior Dimensions.* New York: Raven Press, pp. 269–275.

9

Cancer: A Situational Problem

*A Curriculum for Health Professionals to Teach
Children Whose Parents Have Cancer*

Irene Sullivan, EdD, CSW

This chapter outlines a model curriculum about cancer that health
professionals of various disciplines—physicians, nurses, psychologists, and
social workers—can use to teach children from seven to eleven years of age
whose parents are suffering from cancer.

The statistics on cancer indicate that more people than ever before are living
with cancer. Many of them have children who are also affected by cancer
because the presence of the disease in the parent pervades the family system
and throws it into disequilibrium as parents turn their energies from parenting
toward fighting the disease. Individual roles within the family are disorganized,
disrupting the security of children who expect consistency in nurturing and
discipline from parents.

Established familial communication patterns are interrupted, entangled, and
short-circuited because parents, in their efforts to "protect" children (and
themselves) from further emotional distress, avoid talking with children about
cancer. As a result, children are often left to their own imaginations and conjure
up fantasies more frightening than facts. It has been my experience that children
are capable of providing their own solutions to the situational problems of
cancer when they are provided with relevant information, and with the trust
and support to do so. Parents also benefit when their children are equipped
educationally to deal with situational problems that affect the whole family.

Health professionals, and the resources of the health care setting, are
particularly suited to this educational effort. The professionals who will teach
the course possess, by virtue of their education, a knowledge base that equips
them to teach about cancer as a disease, a relevant part of the curriculum.

60

Health professionals also have the experience of caring for patients with cancer, which provides them with the human knowledge base.

Health professionals are now looking to extend the biomedical model of health education into the biopsychosocial model of education. This curriculum provides them the opportunity to learn from their students, and to experience teaching in that model.

Children who participate will acquire skills that have broad applications. They should acquire the skills to communicate comfortably with their families and with health professionals. They should develop problem-solving skills after learning about cancer as a medical disease, and about cancer as it affects the family. They should come to an understanding of the phases that characterize familial reactions to illness. They should come to an understanding of the changes in roles that affect the equilibrium of the family system, and of the need to reorganize the family during the various phases of disease. They should develop awareness of feelings and attitudes—the family's, the staff's, and their own—through increased empathy; further develop their powers of observation; and learn to respond more effectively to their own needs and to those of their family. Children can thereby develop more positive attitudes about the quality of their own life and the quality of their family life.

THEORETICAL BACKGROUND

Before developing this curriculum, I conducted three literature searches. First, I examined the literature on the social situation, or the context, in which children find themselves when their parents are struck with cancer. It suggested that a cancer curriculum should address two major concerns: the stages and phases of familial reactions to serious illness, and the patterns of familial disorganization, disequilibrium and reorganization in response to illness.

Second, the problem of the children's conceptual view of illness was examined. The literature suggested that, as children grow and mature, and their experiences change, their concepts of illness and causality change also. In order to design a curriculum that children will understand, it is necessary to know the children's view of illness at different ages and stages in their development.

Third, theories of curriculum development were reviewed, and the theoretical models most suitable to the curriculum about cancer were identified. As structured, the curriculum draws on several of the major theories, including (1) Dewey's observation (1938) that a model curriculum should be based on learning from past experiences; (2) Brown's position (1971) that a model curriculum should be based on children's present emotional, cognitive, and behavioral experiences; (3) Tyler's rationale (1949) that a model curriculum should be based on behavioral objectives; and (4) Eisner's stance (1979) that a model curriculum should be based on expressive outcomes and problem-solving objectives. Cognitive and affective taxonomies (Bloom et al 1974; Krathwohl et al 1974) were also used as a reference in examining the learning experiences. Consistent with these theories and models, evaluation is continuous and includes both formal and informal techniques.

Purposes and Goals

The overarching purpose of *Cancer: A Situational Problem* is to enable children to understand that even though their experience of living in a family with a parent who has cancer is painful, it also is an experience from which they can grow by learning to deal with it progressively. By viewing cancer as a situational problem, they can better learn to cope with present and future problems. They can find new, better, and more creative solutions than have been found by others in the past. By viewing cancer as a catastrophic illness that creates a situational problem, they can better learn to value the quality of life, to value themselves, and to value other people as they learn to cope. By viewing cancer as a situational problem that affects thinking, feeling, and action, they can better learn how to bring thinking, feeling, and action together to understand the problem and to develop creative solutions.

Organization

The learning experiences are organized in a sequence whose emphasis shifts from theory to practical application. Appropriate learning activities are structured specifically for active children, to direct their thinking, feeling, and behavior toward understanding present experiences and learning from past experiences. This is consistent with both the cumulative-growth experience and confluent-education models.

The learning activities support each other and represent a progression. First is a warm-up activity to help students become aware of their immediate sense of being in an atmosphere where communication is disrupted (because of cancer in the family) and to become aware that they are not alone in their situation. This activity is planned to enable children with similar experiences to meet, to share, and to support each other.

Next are cognitive, affective, and behavioral learning activities designed to help children deal with their fantasies about cancer and to "discover" cancer cells under microscopes, through the literature, and with audiovisual material. The body and its functions are explored by concrete experiences to enable children to "perceive" what they can otherwise only imagine—the inner workings of the body. Children confront their myths about cancer, understand what we know about the causality of cancer (at their level of understanding), and learn to deal with the uncertainty about causality. Learning experiences are organized to provide children with knowledge about treatments for cancer, with the understanding that the side effects of treatment can make parents feel and look worse, and the reassurance that inside they are still the same parents. Activities follow that enable children to learn from their experiences by thinking, feeling, and acting out the individual and familial problems that arise during the stages and phases of illness, when the family becomes disorganized because of poor communication, redirection of parental energy, and role confusion. Learning experiences are provided to strengthen children's ability to communicate, to expand their view of choices, and to enable them to comprehend cancer as a situational problem with many solutions, some better than others.

The planned learning activities end with the children as "explorers," happy with themselves that they have "discovered" cancer in a new way that will help them to deal with it differently and to teach others about cancer. The learning activities are organized so they may be expanded and developed to meet the needs of new students. They are also designed to be reproduced by the students to teach their family members and peers. Finally, they are organized to include new information about cancer as research and experiences move forward.

A note of caution to educators: These learning experiences, when used sensitively and carefully, will enable children to cope well with their feelings about living with a parent who has cancer. However, the learning experiences will also make children more vulnerable because their emotions will be exposed. Educators need to be alert, sensitive, and supportive of each child. *A learning experience should be modified or omitted if there is reason to believe that any child would be harmed in any way by its use.*

Topics are covered in a planned sequence: the causes of cancer, how professionals search for causes of cancer, where cancer occurs, the treatment of cancer, familial reactions to cancer, and the situational problem of cancer. The first phase enables health professionals to acknowledge that, although children have been "left out" of the diagnosis and treatment phases of their parent's illness, it is important that children understand the basic biology of cancer and have medical information about cancer and its treatment. It is also important that children understand the roles health professionals take in the care of their parents and experience the "hospital" situation. The next phase of activities is planned to enable children to understand what their parents are experiencing physically and emotionally. Subsequent activities are designed to help students understand how cancer creates not only a medical problem, but also a situational problem that disrupts communication, produces an array of (normal) emotions and different behaviors, disorganizes the family system, and so "invades" every part of their emotional, behavioral, and cognitive lives. The activities conclude by enabling students to identify individual situational problems and to arrive at creative solutions with the added dimension of hope.

The sequence, however, is not inviolable, and the modules may be reorganized by teachers to satisfy the particular needs of the children. For example, if the teacher believes that a child will most benefit by beginning with the treatment of cancer and moving from there to the cause of cancer, he or she may do so.

The length of the course is adaptable because the curriculum can be expanded, changed, and modified. It is important, however, that activities include past and present experiences; balance cognitive, emotional, and behavioral domains; and include medical and familial content, allowing students to identify the situational problem of cancer and propose creative solutions.

THE CURRICULUM

Exploring Causes of Cancer

Cancer Explorers (ongoing experience). Health professionals greet students as fellow "explorers" in a new adventure to "discover" cancer. (If possible, students will be given a hospital gown, magnifying glass, or something representative of the hospital.) Throughout the course, health professionals teach children those parts of the course about cancer specific to their expertise (e.g., physicians will help students to discover how cancer is diagnosed). Health professionals assist students to discover the role each health professional plays in exploring causes of cancer and caring for patients with cancer, and assist children to formulate any questions they may have about those roles and about cancer.

Gibberish Warmup. "Gibberish" (adapted from Brown 1971, p. 48) is a warmup activity to help students become more aware of their immediate state of being when the familial communication system is disrupted and they are not provided information, are unable to ask for that information, and are unable to share their emotions about their parent's illness. Students divide into groups of three persons each. Each group is instructed to communicate by using only gibberish (nonsense talk). The groups are then asked to gradually exclude one of the three students from the conversation without using any signs or signals or deciding ahead of time who that person will be. Students are instructed to be aware of whether they are being excluded or included and to be aware of their feelings.

Gibberish Discussion (ongoing experience). Students discuss what they experienced as the "climate" in the gibberish activity (funny, happy, mysterious, fearful, threatening) and why they felt as they did. Students compare those feelings of being included or excluded to their past experiences with cancer and to feelings they think parents, physicians, nurses, and social workers might have. (For example, children may feel rejected, isolated, afraid, while parents may feel protective, powerful, afraid, and health professionals may feel powerful, insecure, anxious.)

Group Fantasy (may follow "Gibberish" or be utilized at any time students need a reminder). "Group Fantasy" (adapted from Brown 1971, pp. 48–49) helps students to understand how lack of information and inability to express feelings produces fantasies that may be either much better or worse than reality. Students divide into seven- or eight-person groups. The members of each group lie in a circle on the floor with their heads toward the center, like the spokes of a wheel. Any student may begin the fantasy, and other students may contribute spontaneously when they are "with" the fantasy. (Health professionals must be careful with this exercise and end the exercise before any fantasies become frightening for any of the students.) Students are asked to sit up, face each other, and report to each other whether or not the fantasies they experienced represented the gibberish they used to converse with each other in the previous exercise. They discuss and compare what they think their behavior might be like after experiencing gibberish and after experiencing their fantasies. Students discuss with each other and with health professionals whether or not they would think, feel, and behave differently if they could feel free to ask questions, express feelings, and share information instead of conversing in gibberish or fantasizing.

Logs. Students keep logs for the whole course. They are encouraged to express themselves in poetry, short stories, and drawings. "Logs" may be used following exercises such as "Gibberish" or "Group Fantasy" and after the "Hospital Tour".

Explorers' Circle. Students sit in a circle. Health professionals discuss the meaning of a "situational problem," as defined by Dewey (1933), and the subject of cancer. Cancer is not just a disease, but a problem—a perplexing, trying situation that involves health professionals, patients, and their families. Participants discuss things explorers do and plan for the unit. "Explorers' Circle" may be used whenever the group needs to be reminded of its central task.

Discussion on Causes of Cancer. Health professionals elicit from students what students think causes cancer. Responses of simultaneity, unrelated sequences of events, the breaking of rules, and other responses that reflect magical thinking and/or notions of punishment, should be encouraged in order to discover the "hidden" thoughts of students about what or who caused cancer in their parents. These may be recorded as hypotheses on chart paper for reference throughout the course. As they are confirmed or refuted, they may be crossed off.

Finding Causes of Cancer. Students will discuss, explore, and write up experiments they think will point out the causality of cancer, or explore various hypotheses. Health professionals may wish to set up experiments and perform some of them at a later time.

Dictionary. Students develop their own dictionary using the vocabulary specific to cancer and, with the assistance of health professionals, analyze the meaning of the words and add to the dictionary throughout the course.

How Health Professionals Search for Causes of Cancer

From One Cell film. Students review, discuss, and analyze with health professionals the film *From One Cell* (American Cancer Society 1978) in order to understand the complex subject of embryonic, regenerative, and degenerative cell behavior. The need to understand cell division in order to understand cancer is explored.

Discovering Cancer Cells. Students compare cancer cells and healthy cells by using a microscope and slides. Health professionals provide individual and group instruction to expand each student's level of understanding of cancer cells and use of the microscope. Students discuss and analyze with health professionals why healthy cells under one microscope do not "catch" cancer or become contaminated by the cancer cells under the nearby microscope. They will "explain" it to themselves in their logs.

Reading About Cancer I. Students read, discuss, and critique appropriate material for their reading level, for example, Chapters 2 and 3 ("From Cell to Man" and "What is Cancer?") in *Cancer* by Silverstein and Silverstein (1973).

How Cells Divide. Students draw pictures of normal and cancer cells, showing the result when normal cells divide to replace dead cells and cancer cells multiply without control. Health professionals assist students with drawing, and ask students to list on the blackboard what they think causes cancer (changes healthy cells to cancer cells).

Reading About Cancer II. Students read, discuss, and critique Chapters 7 and 8 ("Frontiers of Cancer Research" and "Our Dangerous World") in *Cancer* by Silverstein and Silverstein (1973), or other appropriate material.

Questions. Students participate in an exercise, "Questions," adapted from Schleifer (1975 pp. 182–188) to understand the kinds of questions that help them gain the most information. Two students volunteer or are selected to role-play while the other students observe. Student A and student B are instructed to talk to each other for a minute using only questions and no statements. Students discuss how the experience of using only questions feels. Then, student

A asks questions about cancer cells that only begin with "why," and student B answers each question with a statement that begins with "because . . . ." Students reverse roles and then discuss how it feels using "why" questions and "because" answers. Next, student A asks questions about cancer cells that only begin with "how" or "what," and student B answers the questions briefly. Students reverse roles and then discuss how "why" questions and "because" answers differ from "how" and "what" questions and answers. What types of questions provide more information? What types of questions increase feelings of uncertainty?

Questioning Health Professionals. Students question, discuss, and analyze with health professionals their specific roles in the field of cancer. They identify who they can go to for answers to their specific questions about cancer in the hospital, community, and family.

Questions About Causality. Students question, discuss, and analyze with health professionals what we know about the cause of cancer and what we do not know about cancer, using "how" and "what" questions and statements to replace "why" questions. Compare these to questions on the chart.

Critiquing Experiments. Students question, analyze, and critique with health professionals the experiments about the causality of cancer they have begun or written up, and the new experiments related to cancer on which researchers are working.

Blind Walk. Students participate in an exercise, "Blind Walk," adapted from Schleifer (1975 pp. 178–179) to help students deal with confusion or uncertainties about cancer. The blind walk is designed to help students see that when one or more of our abilities, senses, needs, or desires are denied us, we can develop others or we can sabotage ourselves and others by letting the lack of something control us. Students are divided in pairs and instructed to take each other on a blind walk in silence. The length of the walk will depend upon the age and maturity of students. Students A remain blindfolded the whole time, relying on students B to keep them out of trouble, leading them by comfortably holding their arms. Students B let students A know what to avoid, while helping them to feel objects and places, to hear, to smell, and to sense what is around them in the hospital. Students reverse roles in silence. They then discuss in a group with health professionals what they experienced or if they have blinded themselves to the experience. Students and health professionals discuss what uncertainties and confusions they have about cancer, and what discoveries they have made about cancer. They discuss how uncertainties and confusions develop imagination, the beneficial ways imagination can be used, and also the negative result of allowing imagination to control us.

Reading About Cancer III. Students read and discuss Chapter 4 ("Kinds of

Cancer'') in *Cancer* by Silverstein and Silverstein (1973), or other appropriate material.

Identifying Body Parts. Place a transparent model (plastic or wire) of a male and a female with visible, removable parts in front of the room. Students locate and describe the parts of the body within the transparent figures, remove them, and replace them. They are provided with a predrawn form of a male and a female and instructed to draw in the body parts. When completed, they compare their drawings to the transparent models.

Where Cancer Occurs

Locating Cancer Sites. Using models and drawings, students locate cancer sites. They use the terminology in their dictionaries to describe cancer sites in parents and add new words to their dictionaries.

Description and Explanation Vignettes. Students and health professionals compose "description" and "explanation" vignettes in order to explain their parent's illness. (Health professionals will model the vignettes, then have the students do them.) Description vignettes describe the parent's physical behavior caused by the cancer. Explanation vignettes include metaphors to explain the various forms of cancer, body systems, and organ functions.

Treatment of Cancer

Represent Cancer Cells. Using art materials (clay, paper, pencil, scraps), students construct cancer cells. Health professionals discuss and analyze the problems of treating cancer cells, using student models. Health professionals encourage students to identify problems and to pose solutions to treating cancer.

Health Professionals Describe differential treatments for cancer (chemotherapy, X-ray, surgery) and why the treatment to destroy cancer cells often makes parents feel and look worse than before the treatment. Students have an opportunity to question, discuss, and analyze.

Mirrors and Photos. Students look in a mirror and study their appearance carefully. Then they wrap a scarf around their heads to tightly cover their hair and look into the mirror, imagining they have no hair. (Or photos of each student may be photocopied and students may alter the image by covering their hair.) Students will discuss and analyze the ways in which they look different, their feelings about looking different, and the ways in which they feel inside. Does a temporary change in appearance change the way people feel about themselves? Are they basically the same people?

Brainstorm About Feelings. Students "brainstorm" different situations that produce good and bad feelings and result in differential behavior. They analyze how the process and the outcomes may be changed.

Feelings—Behavior Poster. Students think of feelings that produce different behaviors and draw those behaviors on a poster (e.g., if feeling sad, one can sulk in one's room, join a music group, ride a bicycle without looking ahead, or laugh at someone who looks different).

Puppets with Feelings. Students make puppets. The puppets act out emotions that are listed on a card or board (angry, hopeful, hateful, resentful).

Feelings and Hope. Students use puppets to elicit a list of feelings, then write both positive and negative feelings on the blackboard under the heading "Normal Feelings." (This should follow an activity such as "Drawing" or "Inner/Outer Circle.") Health professionals explain that feelings are neutral, not good or bad, and that while we cannot always control feelings, we can control actions. They discuss how feelings make us feel good about ourselves and how they make us feel bad about ourselves when we think they are "bad" feelings instead of normal feelings. Health professionals print HOPE on the blackboard and discuss with students what hope means when connected with feelings.

Understanding Through Color and Images. Students participate in a color-drawing activity (adapted from Schleifer 1975, pp. 180–181) to help them learn about themselves and others through color and images. Students draw one picture (real or abstract) using one color (either red, yellow, or black) in crayon, paint, or colored paper, showing how their parents looked before the illness. Then they draw a second picture, using one of the above colors, showing how parents look after treatment of the illness (no hair, missing limb or partial organ, overweight, underweight, same). Students who wish may share by forming groups composed of other students who used the same colors for the first picture and discuss what the colors mean as they relate to the first drawings. Members of the three different color groups (red, yellow, and black) exchange ideas about what the colors and images mean. Students form groups and repeat the exercise with the second drawings. What do colors and lines tell students about themselves? About their ill parents? What surprised them?

Inner and Outer Circle. Students form two circles (an inner circle and an outer circle) facing a partner. Each student in the inner circle plays the role of child and each student in the outer circle plays the role of a parent responding to his or her child. The students in the inner group tell their "parents" (partners) what they are trying to tell them in their drawings. The students in the outer groups respond to their "children" (partners), first by accepting their feelings and second by providing them with hope and support. The attitude of hope as described by Kubler-Ross (1969) is the basis for the instructions about hope that health professionals provide students. "Children" (partners) will respond to "parents" (partners) by sharing their feelings of hope and support.

Write a Letter. Students write a letter to an imaginary child who has just learned about a parent having cancer. They explain how it feels to be a child whose parent is being treated for cancer, how those feelings may conflict (e.g., one can empathize and feel repulsed; feel frightened that it can happen to you and feel glad it happened to someone else instead; feel sorry for the ill parent and angry at the ill parent because illness interferes with childhood needs), and how feelings make us feel badly about ourselves when we do not accept them as normal reactions to illness. Students draw a picture of one negative feeling that other students also feel, and draw a smiling face to show that negative feelings are normal feelings.

Familial Reactions to Cancer

Resentment Demand, Appreciation (adapted from Brown 1971, p. 43). This activity is to help students get in touch with and direct their immediate resentments to the cancer that is affecting their lives and their parents' lives. Students draw or represent cancer cells (those created earlier in the unit may be used) and concentrate on fantasizing that these are the cancer cells of their parents. (Puppets may be used if needed.) Students take time to think about and voice their resentments ("I resent you. Because of you I cannot. . . ."). Resentments are feelings; they do not have to make sense and are not to be criticized by students or health professionals. After stating their resentments toward the pictured cancer cells, students state their demands of the fantasized parents ("I want you to. . . ."). Students finish the exercise by telling the fantasized parents what the students appreciate (not necessarily like) about the parents. Health professionals discuss with students how it is normal to feel resentment toward an illness that prevents parents from parenting, and how it is better to talk about resentments than to hide them. How do resentments show themselves when we try to hide them?

Hospital Tour (several days). Students take a tour of the hospital to see the equipment that is used to deal with cancer and to discuss that equipment with health professionals. They visit the laboratory and view cytological slides, discuss a biopsy with a physician or a laboratory technician, discuss medications and chemotherapy with oncologists and pharmacists; they visit the pharmacy to see how medications are prepared. They visit the X-ray rooms and discuss X-rays and equipment with technicians; they visit hospital rooms with nurses and social workers and discuss patient care. They see and discuss the medications placed in cups and needles (preferably given to patients, or students can inject dolls). Students use stethoscopes while sitting still and after running in place to experience how activity changes heart rates. They visit the kitchen and plan menus for cancer patients with the nutritionist. They play games with patients in the recreation area. Health professionals let students experience what it is to be a patient, a physician, a nurse, and so forth.

Stages of Death and Dying. Health professionals present stages, as outlined in *On Death and Dying* by Kubler-Ross (1969), allowing time for questions and discussion.

Expression Groups. Students and health professionals divide themselves into five groups. Group I is called "denial"; Group II, "anger"; Group III, "bargaining"; Group IV, "depression"; and Group V, "acceptance." First, students generate a list of descriptive phrases for their group. Then students are asked if they have ever personally experienced any of these. Health professionals enourage students who are shy or feel "stuck." (Groups can either rotate through the stages or share descriptions with other groups.) What was the problem that evoked such feelings? What was the behavior that followed those feelings? Was the outcome good or not so good? Why? Would they do things the same or differently? Health professionals encourage students to understand that it is okay to make mistakes because we can learn from those mistakes and do things differently the next time.

Role Play "Stages." Students write a story together (with the assistance of health professionals) that focuses on a child's concern about a parent who is being treated for cancer, but who is caught in a disruptive familial communication pattern because each family member is at a different "stage." The story is then role-played by students. The primary goal is for students to develop problem-solving skills that will enhance their abilities to:(1) identify the problem situation within the family, (2) generate alternative solutions, (3) evaluate the consequences of alternate solutions, and (4) enable students to acquire new, more productive behaviors. The focus of the role-play situation is on enabling students to explore their own anxieties and communication patterns when discussing illness with parents. It is also intended to provide an opportunity for students to begin to appreciate the concerns and communication patterns that parents use when discussing illness with children. The educational objectives of role play and discussion are formulated to: (1) provide an opportunity for students to begin to appreciate that by understanding stages they can understand why familial communication is disrupted, and (2) provide an opportunity for participants and observers to develop and articulate alternative strategies. Students and health professionals discuss how the stages produce confusion or clarity of thinking, block or open communication, and interfere with or enable problem identification and problem solving. When parents and children are in the same stage, what are their feelings? Behaviors? When they are in different "stages," what are their feelings? Behaviors? What problems arise or are resolved? Can those problems be resolved? In what ways?

Role-Play Mutual Pretense. Students and health professionals participate in activities of "mutual pretense" to enable them to understand how it feels to need to share an important happening with another person and how it feels when one's need to receive affective understanding and cognitive support is prevented by avoidance techniques. This group is instructed to avoid hearing what the designated student wants to share, because they are instructed to show no emotions, and to try to prevent the designated student from showing any emotions. Students and health professionals discuss how feelings and information are affected by mutual pretense. How do we use rituals to avoid emotional communication? Who might take the responsibility to terminate mutual pretense? How? What are the risks? What are the values?

Sentence Completion. Students participate in a "Sentence Completion" exercise (adapted from Brown 1971, p. 44). This may follow the "mutual pretense" activity; groups complete the following sentences, saying them to each member of their group: "I avoid communication with you by. . . ."; "I could communicate with you by. . . ."; "I keep myself from getting involved with you by. . . ."; "I want you to. . . ."

Cave Fantasy. Students participate in this activity (adapted from Brown 1971, pp. 46–47), designed to enable them to relax, get in touch with themselves, and explore doubts and fears about the unknown and about taking risks. Students lie down on the floor, close their eyes, tense every part of their bodies, and at the count of three, relax every part of their bodies as if they were rag dolls. Students are instructed to get in touch with their breathing by taking a deep breath and imagining the fresh air traveling slowly through their bodies down to their toes, then slowly up and out their noses. This exercise is repeated. Students are then instructed to imagine, with their eyes closed, that it is springtime (the sky is blue and the grass is soft and green). They are on a hill with pretty flowers swaying in a soft breeze. They see what turns out to be a dark cave. They examine the opening of the cave, walk into the cave, and see and feel what happens without speaking. After about five minutes, they slowly leave the cave, return to the group, and slowly open their eyes in silence. They sit and draw or paint whatever comes to them. They are asked to share, if they can or wish, their drawings with a partner. Students discuss how it feels to take a risk by walking into a strange situation. Health professionals encourage them to compare the strange situation of an unknown cave to the strange situation of the illness of a parent. Is the unknown frightening? Exciting? Dangerous? Fun? Can it also be beautiful? Enriching? In what way can we make the unknown more enriching than frightening? Do we have to change the cave to do that? Do we have to change ourselves to do that?

Playing Roles. Health professionals explain how they play different roles in their real lives, how we all play different roles voluntarily and involuntarily, what those roles mean to us and to others, how we become "stuck" in obsolete roles, and how we can choose roles and grow from those choices. Students form groups of five or six. Each student makes a list or draws pictures of all the roles they see themselves playing in their family (child, sibling, student, grandchild, basketball player, swimmer, bicyclist . . .). Health professionals encourage students to expand their vision of their roles by giving roles special names, using one sentence to describe themselves (e.g., I am "mothering Millie" because I want to mother all my patients). Students can use the names in cartoon strips (e.g., I am "Snoopy" because I fantasize being powerful like the Red Baron). Students discuss within their groups what names they gave themselves and why—they are encouraged by health professionals to have fun with the names. Health professionals discuss with students how some roles should be temporary, keep people away, draw people together. They discuss how people do not like to take on new roles, and do not like to give up roles, how some roles are felt to be a burden, and the loss of roles may create fears.

Changing Ourselves. This exercise should be modeled for students, using role play, before they begin. Taking turns, students each take a partner. Using puppets, one student in each pair describes a negative role and how he or she would like to change it. The partner observes and makes suggestions to the puppet about how to change his or her role name and change his or her behavior to fit the new role name by discussion and role playing. What happens when roles are changed? Good things? Bad things? How do others respond differently when roles are changed?

Role Vignettes. Students in each group write and act out a vignette about the roles of parents and children and how they change when a parent has cancer. Each character in the vignette is backed by students wearing signs or banners that name all the roles each character plays. Students wearing name signs move behind different characters as those characters take over their roles. (A nurturant mother may look for nurturance from children when she becomes ill; a disciplinary father may want the mother to take over his role when he becomes ill; a child may want to become a "member of the board" within the family system.) When new roles are not accepted by different characters, students wearing those names stand apart. Students who are observers discuss and analyze what would happen if the character who turned down the role accepted the role. Students in the group play it out to see what happens. The audience discusses what the family wants to achieve (family values) and what each character wants to achieve (individual values). Will the change in roles affect family values? Individual values? Should the changes be temporary? When should they be changed? The audience participates in suggesting ways to work out the conflicts about role changes.

Situational Problem of Cancer

Students Discover the Situational Problem of Cancer by creating a painting or drawing (realistic or abstract) with lines, shapes, colors, and textures, that tells a story of their home environment before cancer struck the family, as it is now, and as they would like it to be. From that creation, they write a story or a letter to a fictitious friend that identifies their personal situational problem of cancer, identifies possible choices, describes possible consequences of each alternative, selects an alternative, and justifies their choices in terms of their personal values.

Culminating Activity. Students join hands in inner and outer circles, sing songs, and envision themselves as "explorers" who have "discovered" cancer for themselves, and who will take what they have learned about cancer as a situational problem back to their communities, schools, and families to share their new knowledge. They write down names, addresses, and telephone numbers of students and health professionals with whom they can keep in contact and continue sharing experiences.

Keeping Up Hope. Health professionals share techniques for staying hopeful and help the students to generate a list, e.g., Talk to a friend; identify a supporting adult.

Prepare a Book advising students of what they need to know. Duplicate and bind for all.

A BIBLIOGRAPHY FOR CHILDREN

ALLISON, L. 1976. *Blood and Guts, a Working Guide to Your own Insides.* Boston: Little, Brown, and Company.

KAUFMAN, J. 1975. *How We Are Born, How We Grow, How Our Bodies Work and How We learn.* New York: Golden Press.

LeSHAN, E. 1972. *What Makes Me Feel this Way? Growing up with Human Emotions.* New York: Collier Books.

McGUIRE, L. 1974. *You—How your Body Works.* New York: Platt and Munk.

MOORE, R., AND THE EDITORS OF LIFE. 1962. *Evolution.* New York: Time, Inc.

NOURSE, A. E., AND THE EDITORS OF LIFE. 1964. *The Body.* New York: Time, Inc.

PFEIFFER, J., AND THE EDITORS OF LIFE. 1964. *The Cell.* New York: Time, Inc.

SILVERSTEIN, A., AND V. SILVERSTEIN. 1972. *Cancer.* New York: The John Day Company.

THOMAS, L. 1974. *The Lives of a Cell: Notes of a Biology Watcher.* New York: Bantam Books.

WATSON, J. W., R. E. SWITZER, AND J. C. HIRSCHBERG. 1971. *My Body—How it Works.* New York: Golden Press.

RESOURCES

Printed Materials from American Cancer Society
The Nature of Cancer (Teaching Kit)
Study Guide for the Film, *From One Cell*
Teachers Guide—Grades K–8
Overhead Transparencies from American Cancer Society
"Cell Structure and Function"
"The Nature of Cancer"

Films from American Cancer Society
From One Cell (revised 1978)
Coloring Book from U.S. Department of Health and Human Services
"Hospital Days—Treatment Ways"
N.I.H. Publication No. 82–22085

EVALUATION

Continuous Evaluation. Health professionals actively listen to and observe each student's thinking, emotional, and behavioral processes at work in the class and during the tour of the hospital to evaluate the student's ability to communicate with health professionals and family in new and more adequate ways. They will observe those same processes to evaluate the student's understanding of cancer as a disease and his or her understanding of the illness as it affects the student and the family. They will also observe the student's ability to grasp new concepts, formulate new ideas, risk making mistakes, and learn from past experiences. A key person should keep anecdotal records of each child and cumulatively and periodically review them as a basis for guiding each child. Critical incidents noted by other health professionals should be included in these records.

Formal Evaluation Techniques include the use of oral and written examinations and the use of qualitative and quantitative measurements to evaluate the student's progress and to evaluate the curriculum in meeting students' educational needs.

For example, to assess problem-solving skills, the student may be asked to write a situational problem about cancer and thoughtfully substantiate that a proposed solution will adequately solve the problem. Health professionals evaluate the student's ability to formulate the problem situation, develop a creative solution, and thoughtfully arrive at a conclusion when applying the solution. Through a qualitative form of evaluation, the student is also evaluated on his or her ability to express understanding of his or her situation in a new and more adequate way (talking, writing, dancing, drawing, painting, or acting). When the student's work is adequate, the educator will be able to perceive cues that evidence a balance between cognition and emotions.

The student is also evaluated on his or her ability to consider alternatives, deal with dilemmas, and resolve contradictions in his or her situational problem of cancer. The student is evaluated on the ability to describe, interpret, and evaluate: (1) the causes and treatment of cancer as we know them, (2) the phases and stages of familial responses to illness, and (3) role confusion within the familial system.

Informal Evaluation Techniques include the use of critical narration in a student/teacher interaction in order to evaluate the student, the teacher's way of teaching, and the curriculum.

Conferences with health professionals are held to gain information about the student's ability to integrate the learning experiences and to describe, interpret, and evaluate his or her problem situation. The student is asked to describe feelings, whether of insecurity or confidence, in communicating with health professionals and with family members about the issues of cancer. Finally, the student is asked to discuss the material and methods used in this course to describe whether or not they have been useful.

REFERENCES

AMERICAN CANCER SOCIETY, INC. 1978. "From One Cell." Film. Bloom, B. S., M. D. Englehart, E. J. Furst, W. H. Hill, and D. R. Krathwohl, eds. 1974. *Taxonomy of Educational Objective Handbook I: Cognitive Domain.* New York: David McKay Co.

BROWN, G. I. 1971. *Human Teaching for Human Learning: An Introduction to Confluent Education.* New York: The Viking Press.

DEWEY, J. 1933. *How We Think.* New York: D. C. Heath and Company.

DEWEY, J. 1938. *Experience and Education.* New York: Kappa Delta Pi.

EISNER, E. W. 1977. "On the Uses of Educational Connoisseurship and Criticism for Evaluating Classroom Life." *Teachers College Record* 78(3):345–358.

EISNER, E. W. 1979. *The Educational Imagination.* New York: Macmillan.

KRATHWOHL, D. R., B. S. BLOOM, AND B. B. MASIA. 1974. *Taxonomy of Educational Objectives— Handbook II: Affective Domains.* New York: David McKay Co.

KUBLER-ROSS, E. 1969. *On Death and Dying.* New York: Macmillan.

SCHLEIFER, J., 1975. *Learning Like a Fool.* California: Confluent Educational Development and Research Center.

SILVERSTEIN, A. AND V. SILVERSTEIN. 1972. *Cancer.* New York: The John Day Co.

TYLER, R. W. 1949. *Basic Principles of Curriculum and Instruction.* Chicago: University of Chicago Press.

10

Using Group Process and Therapeutic Metaphor in the Psychosocial Care of Pediatric Cancer Patients and Their Siblings

Amita Jensen, PhD

A group approach, using metaphor, offers many advantages in providing psychosocial care to pediatric cancer patients and their well siblings. Group therapy provides childhood cancer patients with an opportunity to talk with others who know what they are going through; to share their feelings, fears, and frustrations; to ask the questions doctors are frequently too busy to respond to and parents are too frightened to answer; to trade information about procedures and techniques for coping with them; to find out that even with their bald heads, pale faces, and isolation from their prediagnosis life, they are not freaks and they are not alone. A group experience also helps to bring them out of their own occasional self-pity in response to the needs of others (Jensen 1983).

Healthy siblings of pediatric cancer patients are often uninformed and neglected children; including them in such a group educates them as to what their ill siblings have been experiencing and reduces the magnitude of their imagined fears. Their inclusion in the group also affirms that they, along with their ill brothers and sisters, are important. The group experience provides an opportunity for their legitimate resentment and unmet needs to be identified, expressed, and acknowledged by other children in their same situation and by their own ill siblings, who have usually reaped special benefits from being catastrophically ill (Jensen 1983, 1984).

This author's experience in running an ongoing therapeutic support group for pediatric cancer patients and their siblings indicates that family coping with pediatric cancer is tremendously enhanced when siblings are part of such a group. Children as young as eight years old can blend into and benefit from a group that includes adolescents. As the vast majority of pediatric cancer patients, even those with a poor prognosis, have at least one or two years to live from the time of diagnosis, it is important to provide ongoing psychological care for them on an outpatient, as well as on an inpatient, basis. A support group meeting on a regular basis at a hospital, such as "Kids 'n Cancer" at Valley Children's Hospital in Fresno, California, can accommodate both outpatients and siblings, as well as hospitalized patients.

"Kids 'n Cancer" is a hospital-based, peer support and therapy program for inpatient and outpatient pediatric oncology patients and their well siblings. It began in 1983 as part of a doctoral research project on well siblings. The group meets bimonthly for two-hour sessions centering around medical and psychological aspects of living, dying, and being cured of cancer. It maintains a membership of around 15–20 members, about one-half patients and the other half well siblings. The age range is from eight to eighteen years.

Discussions center around members' current experiences, concerns, and questions, as well as around themes chosen by leaders. Frequently discussed issues are ill members' medical conditions and deaths, coping with anger and fear, communicating clearly and directly, discovering personal resources, and using visualization to control pain or cope with anxiety. (For a detailed discussion of this program, see Jensen 1984.)

Naturally, in an ongoing support group of this nature, difficult topics such as death, feeling abandoned, and feeling helpless and overpowered by uncontrollable events arise and need to be confronted. One approach that seems to help both patients and siblings confront these realities and feelings is metaphor: approaching threatening topics indirectly and unconsciously via symbol, imagery, art, and play. After processing anxiety-producing material symbolically, children can then bring as much of the experience into conscious awareness as is safe for them to do at a given time.

This essay describes some uses of therapeutic metaphor employed in Kids 'n Cancer, a children's group formed to help childhood cancer patients and their healthy siblings cope with the stress and disruption of living with that disease.

THERAPEUTIC METAPHOR

Therapeutic metaphor employs symbol, imagery, and allegory to help children approach, confront, and work through anxiety-producing material without bringing it into conscious awareness. Children normally use metaphor on their own to resolve their conflicts and traumas, as can be observed in their play, art, and dreams (Lowenfeld 1967; Millar 1974; Piaget 1962). Art and play therapies have evolved to utilize this natural healing process for adults as well as for children (Axline 1947; Feder 1981; Kramer 1977; Schaefer 1976; Wadeson 1980).

Children respond favorably to the use of metaphor in therapy, as it is nonthreatening and speaks to them in their own language of imagination and play. Adolescents who might normally reject metaphor as childish respond to it with relief and a sense of returning to a safer, less threatening past when they are undergoing the stresses of a life-threatening illness in themselves or in their siblings.

In Kids 'n Cancer, therapeutic metaphor is used in the forms of art, story, and guided imagery to help members become aware of feelings, behaviors, goals, and resources and to help them confront and manage anxiety, anger, pain, hopelessness, and loss. Guided imagery is also used with patients in the group to enhance the effectiveness of their medical treatments and to develop a sense of control and participation in their own treatment and return to health. In addition to the author's own creations, techniques that have been particularly useful have been adapted from the works of Bry (1976), Grinder and Bandler (1981), Houston (1982), Oaklander (1978), Rozman (1976), Simonton, Matthews-Simonton and Creighton (1978), and Stevens (1971).

ART

Using art with a group of children struggling with life-threatening illness, aggressive treatments, and disruption in family and personal life has many benefits. During the initial six-week series that began Kids 'n Cancer's existence, group members were exposed to discussing their illness and feelings openly for the first time; openness was something that neither their parents nor their physicians had encouraged prior to the start of the group. As a result, anxiety among group members was high.

Member anxiety became even higher when the group was unexpectedly confronted at its second meeting with the news that one of its members had suddenly become terminally ill. At that session, leaders placed drawing materials in the center of the room and invited children to draw at any time they wished during the session. Almost every child present picked up materials to draw at some point; this was followed by a noticeable reduction of tension.

Leaders continued the practice of allowing free drawing, and for several weeks thereafter children were observed to reach for drawing materials when discussions turned to the status of the terminal member, to relapse, and to family conflicts—topics which produced obvious anxiety. Drawing appeared to provide either a catharsis (drawings of catastrophes, wars, wild scribbles, or black, ominous objects), or escape (idyllic scenes, flowers, and hearts and teddy bears). It also seemed to provide children with a reduction in anxiety and/or with a distancing from threatening discussions in order to assimilate only what was comfortable at that point in time.

When the terminally ill child died after the sixth session, the group was ready to discuss his death directly, and no member reached for drawing materials at that time. After the discussion of his death, leaders asked children to close their eyes, empty their minds, and just allow a picture representing the meaning of death to present itself to them, then to open their eyes and without a word to draw their picture of death. All of the children were comfortable drawing death. Several commented how good it felt to be able to "get all those feelings out on paper." Others said that they felt "safe" or "peaceful" after completing the drawing and that they were surprised that death didn't seem so scary to them anymore. Only two children drew frightening pictures, and those pictures were useful to leaders in recognizing the special needs and conflicts of those children.

Leaders have continued to use art exercises from time to time in order to assess psychological states of members, to help members approach topics too threatening to discuss openly, and to express feelings. Children have drawn the "worst thing that's happened to you since you or your sibling was diagnosed," as well as any aspect of living with cancer they wished to draw for a booklet they were illustrating for newly diagnosed patients. Both were helpful in analyzing children's fears and major stresses.

Family Drawings (see Oaklander 1978, pp. 26–32) are excellent for assessing family dynamics, as is the ever useful H-T-P Projective Technique (see Buck 1948 and Wenck 1980 for helpful interpretive guidelines).

Drawing "angry" or "hurt" pictures has enabled members to get in touch with and express feelings they have been reluctant to acknowledge or discuss prior to drawing (Oaklander has a discussion of anger pictures on pp. 42–43). When the feeling has been expressed symbolically, children are somehow helped in finding words to describe it.

In selecting and utilizing art projects, as with all other forms of metaphor, timing and interpretation are critical. Assessment projects (H-T-P or Family Drawings) can be done almost anytime. Other projects need to be selected and utilized only when feelings are high, yet remain unidentified or too threatening for children to discuss directly.

Interpreting children's art above and beyond what children feel they have expressed and meant by their work requires some knowledge of standard psychological interpretation of children's art, as well as intuitive sensitivity to particular children in question and the events affecting their lives. Some books that offer excellent guidelines for using and interpreting children's art in therapy are by Di Leo (1973), Kellog (1969), Kramer (1975), Oaklander (1978), and Schildkrout et al (1972). When utilized sensitively and therapeutically, art can provide an excellent vehicle in group therapy for helping children in distress access feelings, discover inner resources for coping, and manage anxiety. It is also powerful in integrating learnings made via guided imagery.

STORY

Selecting, telling, making up, or enacting stories can be a powerful way to tap into unconscious processes of healing for children in distress. Stories often are metaphors for our lives, as we tend to "think of" stories that have relevance to our experiences, feelings, conflicts, or needs for coping with harsh realities.

In Kids 'n Cancer, leaders have used storytelling in three therapeutic ways. In one, children have been asked to remember and then to enact with other group members their favorite fairy tale. Fairy tales encompass all the basic human emotions, and they also confront the question of evil head on. They indicate that life is fraught with severe challenges and difficulties that must be confronted and overcome (Bettelheim 1976). As such, fairy tales offer a rich source of support and metaphoric catharsis for children forced to face and find ways to cope with the evil of seemingly uncontrollable illness and the power of their own tumultuous emotions.

Children's favorite fairy tales often reflect issues children are coping with in their own lives. As such, it is not surprising that the most popular fairy tale among the changing members of Kids 'n Cancer continues to be "Hansel and Gretel." This tale concerns siblings abandoned by weak and uncaring parents, caught up in a nightmare of evil in the form of a witch, with one sibling being imprisoned in a life-threatening situation while the other is forced to look on helplessly as the day of death comes closer and closer, until, despite the odds, they nevertheless manage to overthrow the witch and return home to find that their family life is restored to its former loving state and they can live happily ever after. The popularity of this tale shows how well story provides a metaphor for the emotional experiences of children. Many children in Kids 'n Cancer do feel at some level that their parents have abandoned them by not protecting them from this evil and by not maintaining their previous happy home life.

Enacting their favorite fairy tales enables children to identify with the characters without actually having to discuss their own threatening situations. The drama validates the nature of the struggle they are waging against cancer, provides a justification and catharsis for their own feelings, and provides reassurance that perseverance pays off. They can choose to be the "wicked" characters when they are feeling particularly angry or vengeful, and they can be the "heroic" characters when they feel the need to triumph. After the dramatization has taken place, children are asked how it felt to take the parts they did, or what they would have done if they had acted out other parts of the story. Then children are asked what in the story could be helpful for a child who was in a difficult situation in life. Children will often draw parallels with their own lives and comment on the resources available to the fairy tale characters that they also have available to them. Then they are asked to draw any part of any of the fairy tales enacted that they found particularly powerful. In sharing drawings, children begin to express their own individual feelings, life situations, and resources that relate to the fairy tale.

Another use of story that is effective with a group of children of this nature is to make up a group story. A leader will begin the story with a sentence that could relate to a situation commonly encountered among these children; each child around the circle then adds a sentence or a paragraph to the story, developing an anxiety-provoking situation, then resolving it. A typical story might begin, "Once upon a time, there was a very good little girl who always ate her vegetables . . . " What children will do with that story seems to depend upon their needs of the moment: occasionally they express their desire to rebel (. . ."until one day she suddenly threw them out the window and they accidentally landed on her doctor's head . . . ''); sometimes they express their need for reassurance that goodness prevails (" . . . and Santa heard about her and invited her to the North Pole to live with him''); sometimes it's their need to confront and deal with evil that is expressed (" . . . but then one day a wicked witch who hated good little girls came to her door and sold her mother a bunch of poisoned carrots for soup . . . '') The benefit of telling a group story is that each child gets to express his or her thoughts, feelings, and wishes of the moment. Leaders can use the material to assess children's needs, as well as to introduce some healing or realistic elements into the story that might help children work through their issues.

GUIDED IMAGERY

Guided imagery is therapeutically focused visualization, a directing and interpreting, for specific therapeutic ends, of pictures created spontaneously by the right hemisphere of the brain. In Kids 'n Cancer, guided imagery has been used to assess feelings, problems, and resources; to provide comfort and relaxation; to manage pain and visualize a return to health; to find answers for, confront, and work through problems; to identify goals and visualize achieving them; and to find meaning in suffering and loss. In a gentle or playful way, guided imagery offers these children hope and a sense of control over lives that seem largely out of their control.

Introductory and Diagnostic Imagery Exercises

Guided imagery requires some preparation for its use. It needs to be legitimized in a world dominated by linear, left-brain thinking and a denigration of the "imaginal." Also, children, as well as adults, need to learn that they will get valid answers from largely unconscious and apparently "silly" processes. An easy way to introduce imagery for the first time is by using it as simple imagination. Children in a group can close their eyes and just imagine themselves on their own streets in front of their own houses. Then they can imagine that a cute puppy dog comes running up to them. They can make friends with this puppy and interact with it however they wish for a few moments, enjoying themselves and the dog. Then they can say goodbye and watch the puppy dog go cheerfully on its way. Children learn in an exercise like this that they can all use and get something from imagery. They also learn about their own unique processes when they compare their puppy dogs with everyone else's. No one's dog is ever the same, and how each dog reacts with each child reveals what that child feels about dogs and about reacting to new people and new situations.

Children can also discover how their bodies are actually affected by imagery, by having them close their eyes and imagine going into a grocery store and coming up to a pile of wonderful oranges—seeing the rich, juicy, orange fruit, smelling that distinctive orange smell, feeling the oranges, even feeling the oil from the oranges rub off on the hands, then cutting open a particularly delicious-looking orange, biting into it and tasting its fresh, cool pulp, feeling its juices running down the throat—then moving over to a counter of lemons, once again appreciating them with all of the senses, picking up and then cutting one in half and plunging it into the mouth, tasting and smelling the lemon, feeling juice squirt in the mouth and run down the throat. Children love the way their mouths pucker, and this exercise provides an impressive argument that imagery has real effects on the body, which is important in using imagery for pain control or to enhance healing.

Another easy and revealing use of imagery as simple imagination is Stevens' "Motorcycle" exercise (Stevens 1971, pp. 154–155), which helps children get in touch with their power and way of operating in the world. Oaklander's "Rosebush Identification" (Oaklander 1978, pp. 32–33) is also an effective introductory exercise to use with children. It shows how they perceive their health, their environmental support, and their resources for coping.

Having group members introduce themselves as the animal they would most like to be provides leaders with excellent assessment information via metaphor. Each child is asked to say what he or she is and describe him or herself. Then they are to state what the most wonderful thing about being this animal is; what it most needs in its life; what it most likes, fears, and hates; how it feels about people; and what it would wish for if it could have any wish in the world come true. Animals selected are remarkably revealing of personalities (even when it is "a snake that lives in the grass"). Much can be learned about how children perceive themselves, what they feel about their lives, and what their relationships are like with their siblings.

Going Deeper: Relaxation and Suggestive Language

The foregoing simple uses of imagery can be done with very little preparation of children. When leaders want to use imagery that taps into deeper layers of unconscious processes, it is wise to proceed only after rapport has been gained with children. It is also wise to build on the imaginative experiences of group work, introducing deeper types of guided imagery only after other forms of metaphor have been experienced and enjoyed. Any particular imagery exercise, of course, should be tailored to precise therapeutic goals and be used only when group conditions are conducive to a relaxed, nonlinear exploration of issues. When group members are agitated, imagery won't work until some of their excess tension has been discharged. For that reason, in Kids 'n Cancer, imagery exercises are sometimes preceded by movement, sound, or art exercises.

A relaxed, receptive mental state is necessary for deeper work with imagery, so children are led through relaxation techniques for a few minutes prior to beginning the imagery itself. As imagery is an inner experience, it is helpful to draw children's attention inward, to their breathing, their bodies, their thoughts, and then to a special, pleasant place that they like to visit. Some relaxation and focusing techniques that work very well with this group of children include Stevens' "Breathing into the Body" exercise (Stevens 1971, p. 260), Jacobsen's Progressive Relaxation (see Samuels and Samuels 1975, p. 106), and exercises devised by Kravette (1979) and Benson (1975). Bry (1976), Rozman (1976), Shorr (1977), Vaughn (1979), and Gawain (1982) also describe useful ways to induce a relaxed, attentive state conducive to effective imagery.

Also important in achieving success with imagery work is instilling expectations of success, of learning, and of delight in the workings of the inner mind. Excellent suggestions for inducing positive expectations can be found in Grinder and Bandler (1981) and in Francuch (1981).

What makes for a powerful imagery experience once children move into it in a relaxed state are specific, sensual, vivid suggested images. It helps to have children move into the experience with all of their senses: seeing what's around them; smelling the air; feeling the ground beneath their bare feet, or the sun beaming down warmly on their shoulders, or their bodies plunging into a refreshing mountain pool; hearing the sounds of waves, or birds, or the breeze blowing through the trees; even tasting the saltiness of the sea air on their lips or of Grandma's famous pumpkin pie. The more vivid and sensual the imagery is, the more real the experience is to children, the more it will transport them from their present situations to healing ones, and the more their bodies will participate in and reflect the experience.

Imagery for Comfort

Relaxation techniques, positive expectations, and specifically soothing images by themselves can do much to relieve anxiety in distressed children, both within a group setting and within an acute hospital setting. Children find safety in being able to regain control in panicky situations by focusing on and controlling their own breathing and then in being able to "escape" the terrifying situation by retreating vividly in their minds to a special safe place. A simple focus on breathing, along with the stated expectation that breathing was indeed possible, has calmed a leukemic child who was hemorrhaging in the throat and allowed him to be able to breathe. A similar focus on breathing, followed by imagery transporting them to their own bedrooms or Disneyland, has helped many children manage their terror during bone marrow aspirations.

Imagery which transports them back to earlier, happier periods of their lives can be of great comfort to patients and siblings living with the prolonged anxiety and disruption of cancer. Children experiencing such prolonged stress will often display symptoms of regression, and such exercises as these provide children with an opportunity to regress asymptomatically.

One exercise that has provided children with a return to a safer past and also given them a greater appreciation of themselves, their resources, and their joys is "Childhood Regression." Children as young as seven seem to be able to "return to themselves at age five." This exercise requires relaxation and imagery that will transport children away from the present moment. Children are asked to relax, feel like they are lying on their backs on a nice, sunny day watching clouds go by, then watching autumn leaves blowing on a tree, then following one particularly beautiful leaf as it is blown high into the sky, higher and higher until it comes quite unexpectedly to a golden castle shimmering in the sky, then into a room in the castle with a book in it with a full sensory description of today's activities in it, then leafing back through the pages, moving back through time, all the way back to a long, long time ago when they were four or five years old, to the perfect day for making new learning about themselves. Then they are asked to visualize themselves in detail as they are at that age, noticing their hair, its color and cut, their eyes, their mouth, how they are dressed, whether they have on shoes or not, what they are engaged in doing this day. They are asked to look at the expression in their eyes and see what it is and answer the question, "What kind of a child am I—quiet, shy, boisterous, rowdy, happy, worried, etc.?" They are asked to explore their world and what they most love doing in it, re-experiencing engaging in their most loved activities with all of their senses and noting how their bodies feel and their faces look when they do. Then they are asked to allow their present self to enter the scene and meet their younger self, becoming friends, allowing the older self to say that it appreciates and values the little child, interacting with it for awhile. Before leaving any such positive imagery, children are always instructed that they can return to this time, place, and experience any time they want to take a few minutes to relax and come back here.

The comfort and learning from this experience is profound, especially if children have the opportunity to move from the imagery experience out into the world all alone, taking their five-year-old with them on a walk, and for 15–30 minutes just allowing their inner child to show them his or her world, with all of its wonders and joys, doing whatever that little child most wants to do. The "older self" is to protect the younger self and make sure that he or she doesn't get hurt in any way. Children will often return to this experience, or allow themselves to engage in those earlier activities, as a way of loving themselves when they are feeling lonely, bored, or tired of coping with the realities their "older selves" have to continue to confront day after day.

Imagery for Controlling Pain and Assisting in Healing

Imagery can invoke the power of the mind to create a desired result. It definitely has an effect on perceived pain. Some researchers (Samuels & Samuels 1975; Simonton et al 1978) believe that imagery can effect healing as well, utilizing the placebo effect. But even if it can't make a child's cancer go away, the use of imagery does give children a sense of participating in their own treatments and of having some control over their bodies and over what's happening in them. This sense of control seems directly related to children's abilities to make good psychological adjustments to their illnesses.

In using imagery to affect the body, relaxation is important, and it can be achieved even with terrified children if they can stop screaming long enough to start breathing into their pain. Children can imagine drawing air into their bodies and sending it directly to the area of pain, then blowing the pain out with the exhalation. They can breathe just as deeply and rapidly as they need to to keep blowing out all of the pain. It's remarkable how rapidly the pain gets "blown out" in this manner. Normally children only have to take three or four rapid breaths before they begin to slow their breathing down because the pain is being controlled by it. This focus on the breathing, adjusting it to the intensity of the pain, removes children from their terror, provides them with a sense of control, and results in deeper, slower breathing, which is naturally relaxing.

Another way children can work with pain that is not of such terrifying proportions is to close their eyes and focus on the pain, becoming acutely aware of it. They are to focus on and describe out loud what kind of pain it is, how strong it is, exactly which parts of the body are affected by it, what shape or shapes it has, how big it is, what color it is, what texture it has, and what is happening to it as they keep watching it. If they notice any changes in it, which almost invariably happens, they are asked to see if they can increase the pain for a moment, to make it grow and become worse. Then they are asked if they can move it to another place in the body, or change its shape or color. Subconsciously they are beginning to realize that they have some control over this force which heretofore they felt had total control over them. Finally they are asked to see if they can reduce the pain by letting it go in some way. Here, breathing the pain out a little bit with each breath seems to work well. In most cases, the pain will simply disappear at this point. When it doesn't entirely leave, children can be asked to become the pain and to describe themselves. What are they like? What do they do to the person who has them? What is their attitude as this pain? What message do they, as the pain, have to give the children who are receiving it? Children can engage in a dialogue with the pain, asking it what it wants from them, and telling it how they feel about the pain and what they want from it. Often unmet needs and conflicts will emerge in such a "symptom dialogue," both for siblings with psychosomatic symptoms and for patients with pain from their cancer. Acknowledging the ignored feelings, or negotiating a compromise, will often relieve the pain. If not, the pain can be talked to with appreciation for its function in alerting the child to the need for action, but told that the child is well aware of the problem and is doing everything that can be done to correct the problem, so the pain is no longer needed and is requested to leave at this time.

The use of imagery to visualize the physical condition of the body, the effectiveness of chemotherapy or radiation therapy in combatting cancers, the impact of a fully activated immune system destroying cancer cells, and a return to perfect health, has been well described by Simonton et al (1978), Samuels (1975), and Bry (1976). Imagery for healing will thus not be discussed here except to say that children can use this imagery very effectively and that once again specificity, vividness, and full sensory detail appear to enhance the power of the imagery employed. A relaxation technique that is particularly effective if used prior to this healing imagery is Schultz' Autogenic Therapy (*see* Samuels pp. 223–226), which demonstrates the power of the mind in creating changes of temperature and warmth in the body as it induces a relaxed state. Children can feel for themselves that the imagery is already working, thus enhancing their positive expectations about the potential for healing.

Processing and Integrating the Guided Imagery Experience

The learnings gained from guided imagery can be processed either symbolically or verbally. Sometimes drawing part of the imagery experience can be helpful to children in expressing the feelings associated with it, or in claiming the healing power of the imagery. Likewise, acting out the drama of the imagery experience can help children integrate its messages.

In Kids 'n Cancer, children are also given the opportunity to process imagery experiences consciously, should they choose to do so. Discussions are held after each exercise to determine what children experienced, what their feelings were about the experience, and what they may have learned about themselves or about the experience of living with cancer. In working verbally with imagery, it is important to find out what the images mean to each child and to work within his or her meanings. If a child has had a frightening or frustrating experience, the child can be guided back into the experience, equipped with some appropriate protection or strategy for resolution, and then helped to confront and overcome the difficulty encountered. Other group members listening to this re-entry can often provide ideas for both protection and for dealing with the problem situation. In engaging in this re-entry, both the working child and the supportive group members gain awareness of their abilities to cope with and to overcome difficulties, even when they may be frightened at the time. Certainly, however, if a child balks at some fearful imagery, he or she should never be forced to confront it, but can be helped to find ways to protect himself or herself from being hurt by it in the future. Children's defenses normally come to their rescue; if they are too threatened by any experience, they will simply shift their attention to other matters.

CONCLUSION

Therapeutic metaphor allows children living with cancer to explore and resolve issues and feelings on an unconscious level that seem overwhelming to their conscious ego. Its use appears to reduce anxiety sufficiently for children to begin to deal with their feelings on a conscious level. The differences in the psychological adjustment and behavior of both patients and well siblings in Kids 'n Cancer as a result of a group experience relying heavily on the use of therapeutic metaphor has been significantly positive (Jensen 1983). In addition to helping children find new resources for coping with harsh realities, metaphor also gives them an opportunity for fun, laughter, and magic in the midst of tragedy—a chance to transcend.

REFERENCES

AXLINE, V. 1947. *Play Therapy*. New York: Ballantine Books.

BENSON, H. 1975. *The Relaxation Response*. New York: William Morrow and Co.

BETTELHEIM, B. 1976 . *The Uses of Enchantment: The Meaning and Importance of Fairy Tales*. New York: Knopf.

BUCK, J. 1948 "The H-T-P Technique: A Quantitative and Qualitative Scoring Manual" *Clinical Psychology Monographs,* 5:1–120.

BRY, A. 1976 . *Visualization: Directing the Movies of Your Mind*. New York: Barnes & Noble Books.

DI LEO, J. 1973 . *Children's Drawings as Diagnostic Aids.* New York: Brunner/Mazel.

FEDER, E. AND B. FEDER. 1981. *The Expressive Arts Therapies.* Englewood Cliffs, N.J.: Prentice-Hall, Inc.

FRANCUCH, P. 1981. *Principles of Spiritual Hypnosis.* Santa Barbara, CA: Spiritual Advisory Press.

GAWAIN, S. 1982. *Creative Visualization.* New York: Bantam.

GRINDER, J. AND R. BANDLER 1981. *TRANCE-formations: Neuro-Linguistic Programming and the Structure of Hypnosis.* Moab, Utah: Real People Press.

HOUSTON, J. 1982. *The Possible Human.* Los Angeles: J.P. Tarcher.

JENSEN, L.A. 1983. *Siblings of Children with Life-Threatening Illness: An Assessment of Psychological Reactions and an Approach to Treatment .* Ann Arbor: University Microfilms International.

JENSEN, L. A. 1984. "Kids 'n Cancer, An Innovative Treatment Program for Pediatric Oncology Patients and Their Siblings." Miami: Third Annual Conference of International Association of Pediatric Social Workers, November.

KELLOG, R. 1969. *Analyzing Children's Art .*Palo Alto, CA: National Press Books.

KRAMER, E .1975. *Art as Therapy with Children.* New York: Schocken Books.

KRAMER, E. 1977. *Art Therapy in a Children's Community.* New York: Schocken Books.

KRAVETTE, S. 1979. *Complete Relaxation.* Rockport, MA: Para Research.

LOWENFELD, M. 1967. *Play in Childhood.* New York: John Wiley.

MILLAR, S. 1974. *The Psychology of Play.* New York: Jason Aronson.

OAKLANDER, V. 1978 .*Windows to Our Children.* Moab, Utah: Real People Press.

PIAGET, J. 1962. *Play, Dreams and Imitation in Childhood.* New York: Norton.

ROZMAN, D. 1976. *Mediation for Children.* Millbrae, CA: Celestial Arts.

SAMUELS, M. AND N. SAMUELS. 1975. *Seeing with the Mind's Eye: The History, Techniques and Uses of Visualization.* New York: Random House.

SCHAEFER, C., Ed. 1976. *Therapeutic Use of Child's Play.* New York: Jason Aronson.

SCHILDKROUT, M., I. SHENKER, AND M. SONNENBLICK. 1972. *Human Figure Drawings in Adolescence.* New York: Brunner/Mazel.

SHORR, J. 1977. *Go See the Movie in Your Head.* New York: Popular Library.

SIMONTON, O.C., S. MATTHEWS-SIMONTON AND J. CREIGHTON. 1978. *Getting Well Again: A Step-by-Step, Self-Help Guide to Overcoming Cancer for Patients and Their Families.* Los Angeles: Jeremy P. Tarcher.

STEVENS, J. 1971. *Awareness: Exploring, Experimenting, Experiencing.* Moab, Utah: Real People Press.

VAUGHN, F. 1979. *Awakening Intuition .* Garden City, NY: Anchor.

WADESON, H. 1980. *Art Psychotherapy.*New York: John Wiley.

WENCK, L.S. 1980. *House-Tree-Person Drawings: An Illustrated Diagnostic Handbook.* Los Angeles: Western Psychological Services.

11

Cancer: A Curriculum for Well Siblings of Pediatric Cancer Patients

by Irene Sullivan, CSW, EdD

At the request of the Social Work Department of Memorial Sloan-Kettering Cancer Center, I designed a curriculum about cancer that is being used by physicians, social workers, psychologists, nurses, recreation therapists and teachers to educate well-siblings from 6 to 17 years of age of pediatric cancer patients. The aim of the curriculum, "Cancer: A Curriculum for Well-siblings of Pediatric Cancer Patients," is to provide children with the information about cancer that would enable them to understand better and to cope well with their experiences of living in a family with a brother or sister struck with a catastrophic illness.

The need for such a curriculum was evident almost immediately when the author interviewed, at Memorial Sloan-Kettering Cancer Center, the parents and nine-and eleven-year-old brothers of a sixteen-year-old boy suffering the last stages of cancer. The parents expressed their concern that their two healthy sons had little knowledge about the disease and about the treatment provided to their ill son, and also expressed their concern that they themselves were too emotionally and physically involved with their ill son to provide information that would help their sons cope with an illness that affected the whole family. The ill son also expressed concern for his brothers, and agreed with his parents that a course about cancer would benefit the whole family. The two brothers, when asked about their sibling's illness, thought their brother "probably caught the disease when he caught a large fish in a stream close to home and put his arm all the way into its mouth." The brothers described how they "fished in the same stream, but only put their fingers in the mouth of fishes to remove the hook." They were concerned that the water did not look too clean, and that sometimes it seeped into their house. When asked by the author if they would like more information about cancer they responded enthusiastically.

Children are surviving childhood cancer, when only a generation ago there were few survivors. The literature that once focused on young patients, their siblings and parents facing the death of the sick child, or surviving that death, changed its direction to concentrate on young patients and their parents living with a threatening illness. Clinical observations and retrospective studies that include the well sibling, living in a family with a brother or sister surviving cancer, are beginning to emerge in the literature. But instead of focusing on adaptability of the well sibling, the literature emphasizes pathology. There is a glaring absence of prevention strategies that educate siblings to cope well with all the problems involved with having a brother or sister sick with cancer.

Well siblings are often left with little, or confusing, information about the cancer that dramatically affects their lives. Knowledge about cancer, its treatment, the resultant physical and emotional effects, and adaptive coping strategies, is not easily available to well siblings. Childhood cancer is not a predominant disease, and the specific cause is still unknown. School textbooks provide outdated and sparse information about cancer, and many books still call it a "killer disease." Television programs concentrate on adult audiences by urging viewers to avoid cancer by not smoking, drinking, or breathing contaminated air. Well siblings are usually excluded from family conferences when the diagnosis of cancer and the regimen of treatment is first discussed. Children are "boarded out," or left with relatives and friends when parents turn all their energies toward care of the sick child in the early stages of diagnosis and hospitalization. Communication with well children is often by telephone, often providing only little or confusing bits of information by parents who are emotionally overwhelmed and physically exhausted in caring for the sick child. Well siblings feel alone and anxious as they struggle with emotional and developmental issues with which they hesitate to burden parents.

A lack of information, lack of communication, and consequently a lack of understanding of the sibling's illness may produce guilt feelings in well siblings too young to understand fully how illness is caused. Cognitive confusion can produce feelings of anxiety that somehow the well sibling caused his brother or sister to become sick.

Treatment of the disease by chemotherapy, surgery and radiation may produce side effects such as temporary loss of hair, lethargic feelings, moodiness, nausea and vomiting, perhaps the loss of a limb. The sibling looks different and behaves differently than she or he did before becoming sick. The sibling relationship becomes strained when the ill sibling is not prepared for the drastic physical changes and intense emotional drama that is played throughout the family system. Hearing about, or witnessing, the painful procedures the sick child endures is frightening. Well siblings become fearful of their own vulnerability, and anxious about the threat to the sick child's life.

Emotional realignment, in which a triad of mother, father and sick child is formed, leaves the well sibling feeling rejected, anxious, angry and lonely. Normal jealousy among siblings increases in response to the special privileges and extra attention given to a sick brother or sister, as parents become over-protective of the sick child, and less tolerant and more demanding of the well child. The resentment becomes bi-directional when the sick child feels angry at the sibling for being well. Caring for each other also emerges, but often the well sibling takes on too much responsibility as parental expectations increase, or reaction formation is used as a defense.

Feelings of sibling rivalry, low self-worth, anxiety, fear, shame, embarrassment, guilt, loneliness, sadness, anger, resentment, abandonment, rejection, and isolation often emerge, with resultant symptoms as children become more vulnerable to somatic illness and accidents.

Peer relationships become strained at a time well siblings need more support. Friends withdraw, leaving the well sibling feeling more alone to struggle with an overwhelming and incomprehensible set of events. Peers often tease and make fun of the sick child, placing the well sibling in a position of protecting a brother or sister, while feeling angry, embarrassed, ashamed and "different."

The well sibling is concerned that the family is different from other families who do not have a child with cancer. Parents are concerned about their well children, and are asking for assistance to bring the energy of the family system into a better balance to the benefit of all members of that system.

Cancer is a devastating disease, not only because it is one of the leading causes of death in the United States; but because it separates well children from parents and ill siblings, often leaving well siblings isolated emotionally and physically and deprived of education about cancer that would enable children to cope in a better way with living in a family struck by cancer.

LITERATURE REVIEW

The use of various methods of education to facilitate the optimal coping of family members affected by cancer is only recently being recognized by health professionals and educators as a primary prevention strategy. Educational approaches have been found to be useful when designed for specific populations within the family system.

Adams-Greenly and Moynihan (1983) maintain that an individualized educational approach is useful when teaching a parent to assess a child's cognitive abilities and emotional responses to cope with the parent's illness. This enables the parent to clarify the child's misconceptions about causality with age-appropriate explanations. Books are offered to the parent for their own intellectual mastery of the disease. Age-appropriate books are also provided for the parent to read to their children. McCollum (1974) notes the value of teaching parents effective ways to seek information constructively about their child's disease. Parents are also taught to assess the developmental status of their child. Preparing questions in advance, the parent can make optimal use of conferences with the physician, and accommodate the treatment regimen to the developmental status of the child. Duberley (1974) points out that education of the sick child should begin upon admission to the hospital. Assessment of the child's level of comprehension, and the way in which the child uses speech and language, makes it easier to find the words he will understand when a member of the hospital staff tells the child what is likely to happen to him in the hospital. This allows the child to ask questions about the things that worry him.

Sourkes (1980) points to the cognitive confusion of the well sibling, and offers valuable insight into the two views the sibling often holds about how a brother or sister's illness was caused. One view stems from the medical information heard from parents and doctors. The other view is the sibling's own "private version," often unarticulated, but to which he/she clings with tenacity. Cognitive confusion occurs when a child applies simultaneity or sequence of an overwhelming and incomprehensible set of events to cause. Magical thinking surfaces to make sense of those emotionally charged events. The visibility or invisibility of the disease and the treatment contributes to the cognitive confusion. Thus, the medical view must be reiterated many times during the illness. In everyday situations, a child can be shown that simultaneity or sequence does not necessarily imply cause. Koch, Herman and Donaldson (1974) stress the need for parents to state explicitly that nothing anyone did, said, or thought was responsible for the disease.

Spinetta (1978, 1981) points out that active and continued communication is essential because siblings need to become aware of, actively express, and resolve issues and feelings related to the disease and its treatment. An open family system of communication enables members to grow closer together. He cautions, however, that a forced openness, too soon for some families, can be destructive. Gogan and Slavin (1981) maintain that a sense of constraint within the family system continues for many years when siblings try to raise questions about the subject of their brother's or sister's illness. A lack of information, lack of communication, and consequently poor understanding of the sibling's illness, may produce guilt feelings in well siblings too young to understand fully how illness is caused, and believe they are somehow responsible for the disease. Bingen (1973) reports that siblings of children who died with leukemia feel responsible for the sibling's death, and are often preoccupied with inner fantasies of death and fearful that they will be next. Many express anger at the parents who allowed the siblings to become ill. Heffron, Bommelaere, and Masters (1979) point out that siblings modify their behavior considerably when they have a more complete understanding of leukemia and its management. Kramer (1984) contends the lack of information commences when the well children are not included in the initial family conferences and the primary information is given about the disease and its treatment. Well siblings cannot easily visit the hospital, or are "boarded out" at the homes of relatives and friends. Gaps in information prevail because communication between parents and well siblings is often carried out by telephone, adding more stress to the physical and emotional separation caused by parents busy at the hospital, and feeling overwhelmed themselves.

Cunningham, Betsa and Gross (1973) maintain that siblings feel some degree of mystery, shame and embarrassment attached to the illness. Children are concerned that their families are different from other families. Albin, Binger, Stein, Kushner, Zoger and Middelson (1971) point out that siblings are angry because of the disruption of the family as a result of the disease, and this reaction is normal.

Caiars, Clark, Smith and Lansky (1979) note that similarities between siblings and patients are striking in their anxiety levels about their own health, and both groups express negative feelings about their body images. Lindsay and MacCarthy (1974) state that psychosomatic symptoms occur as the child's preferred reaction to stress. The child may become more vulnerable to infections as a way to obtain the concern of the parents. Behavior may evidence a need for punishment and for attention as the sibling becomes more accident prone. Binger (1969) points out the more severe reactions that follow the death of a sibling are enuresis, headaches, poor school performance, school phobia, depression, severe anxieties and persistent abdominal pains.

Emotional realignment in the family system places a strain on relationships within the family. Gogan and Slavin (1981) point out that normal jealousy among siblings can be heightened in response to special privileges and extra attention given to the sick brother or sister, especially when they do not understand the seriousness of the patient's situation. Siblings often believe that the patient has been overprotected, and that the parents have demanded less from him or her than the siblings. Kagen-Goodheart (1977) maintains that the resentment felt by siblings is bidirectional when ill siblings are angry at their brothers and sisters for being well. Sourkes (1980), on the other hand, notes that positive caring can be bidirectional, and often the children's most adaptive means of coping. Lindsay and MacCarthy (1974) point out that feelings of resentment might be turned into caring by the costly defense of reaction formation.

Kramer (1984) reports further on the negative aspects of cancer that affects sibling relationships. Well siblings feel guilty because they are healthy and enjoy unrestricted play activities while the ill child is homebound or hospitalized.

They feel potential guilt over the possibility, for example, of exposing the immunosuppressed leukemic child to a complicated secondary illness. The therapeutic regimen changes the sick child's personality and physical appearance. Loss of hair due to radiation and chemotherapy is a most disturbing change, but substantive gains and losses in the sick sibling's body weight are also very upsetting. Hearing about or witnessing the painful procedures the ill child undergoes is frightening, as it confirms the threat to the child's life, and raises anxiety over the sibling's own vulnerability to illness. Medication results in lethargy and moodiness, often straining sibling relationships. Social activities become restricted when the illness and the therapeutic regimen prevent families from doing things they used to do together. The effects of cancer and its treatment often strain the relationship with peers. Some friends become more supportive, but others often withdraw, and, sadly, some peers will tease the ill child who looks different.

Kramer (1984) maintains that there are positive aspects of the effects of the leukemic illness when healthy children express feelings of empathy and love and want to care for and protect the ill sibling. Well siblings mature from the experience, develop greater inner strength, become more tolerant of others, develop a more positive attitude, value good health, and make the most of each day. Family relationships become more cohesive as relationships are more highly valued.

Cain, Fast and Erickson (1969) point to the complexity of the issues that emerged from their study of children's disturbed reactions to the death of a sibling. The issues include affect, cognition, belief systems, superego functioning and the object relationships of the well sibling. The distortions are intertwined with the dynamics and structure of the family. They may significantly involve the extended family as well as the child's peers, and even his general neighborhood and community. They include characteristics of the sick child and the developmental level of the well sibling, with particular emphasis upon the child's cognitive capacity to understand illness and death; the availability to the child of the parents and various substitutes; and major concurrent stresses upon the child and his family. The effects on the child undergo constant developmental transformation and evolution. Prevention opportunities almost automatically involve professional people from several disciplines.

In several ways, hospitals are providing a natural milieu for educating family members to cope with the effects of cancer. Adams-Greenly and Moynihan (1983) point out the various educative opportunities available in the hospital setting to support the family adequately, and prepare a young child to cope with the serious illness of a parent. Preparation for the visit must take into account the age of the child, the acuity of the parent's condition, and sociocultural factors. Interpretation of the parent's medical status must first address the child's observations. Clarification is relevant that sickness is the cause for the change in behavior and activity, not anything the child has thought, said, or done. "It is important to emphasize that the sick parent does not want to be away from the child and is hospitalized only because it is necessary." Simple and specific explanations of kinds of hospital equipment and the helpful role they play helps young children become familiar and comfortable with the hospital environment. Equipment such as intravenous tubing, gauze and other supplies given to the child helps to elicit questions and concerns. Encouraging the child to sit on the parent's bed, touch, and hug the parent, helps to normalize the situation. After the visit, the child can draw a picture which may serve to clarify the experience and resolve any misinformation or fears the child may have. "When there is a major body change in the patient, such as might be caused by radical surgery or a dramatic weight loss, young children may have difficulty integrating their perceptions with their previous knowledge of the parent. It is helpful to discuss the children's fears and to reassure them that this is still their parent, who loves them and wants to see them."

Kagen-Goodheart (1977) notes the value of encouraging well siblings to visit hospitalized sick brothers and sisters so they do not build up fantasies about the ill child. It also enables them to see the hospital in a better perspective and to ask questions themselves of doctors and nurses. Lindsay and MacCarthy (1974) state that frequent visiting by the well sibling will give the parents a chance to bring up any problems they may have. Munson (1978) finds hospital visiting an opportunity for the health team to evaluate the sibling subsystem for an overprotective family pattern, which can lead to severe problems for siblings. Overprotectiveness encourages fantasies of responsibility for the illness as well as concerns for their own well-being. If the parents feel secure about answering young children's questions about the illness, an opportunity for the children to discuss their concerns with medical personnel should be provided. Kagen-Goodheart (1977) points out that the expectations of the patient's siblings are that all will go on as before once the patient has returned from the hospital.

Kramer (1984) offers suggestions for providing educational support to well siblings in the hospital setting. They include the inclusion of the siblings at the initial family conferences, arrangements for follow-up teaching sessions in the hospital or outpatient clinic at convenient times for siblings, and the use of teaching strategies, such as slide presentations of procedures (e.g., lumbar punctures, IV chemotherapy) and use of puppet play to show how the procedure equipment is used. Intervention strategies would include an initial family assessment about the well children at home, sibling involvement in the care of the ill child, the development of an emotional-support sibling network, and encouragement of an open family communication system.

This review of the literature has revealed several major concerns about the information that children need in order to cope with the problem of living with a sibling who has cancer. One concern involves information about the nature of cancer, the types of cancer, the diagnoses of cancer and the causation of cancer. Another concern involves the treatment of cancer and the effects of that treatment. The affective/behavioral, and cognitive responses to childhood cancer are relevant, not only to the nature of cancer and its treatment, but also to the way in which family relationships are affected by childhood cancer, and to the way in which peer relationships are affected by childhood cancer. All of these concerns as evidenced in the literature suggest the knowledge base for "Cancer: A Curriculum for Well-siblings of Pediatric Cancer Patients."

RATIONALE

The curriculum has been designed to enable well siblings of pediatric cancer patients to understand more broadly and deeply the meaning of the concept of cancer and its effect on well siblings. Content has been organized to provide well siblings with medical information about cancer and its treatment, using as a resource guide "The Bibliography for Educators." Sequential development of content provides information about the emotional and behavioral patterns of well siblings, using the "Literature Review" section as a resource guide. The content concludes with the encouragement of well siblings to support each other in identifying problem situations; reviewing relevant medical information, patterns of emotions, and behavioral patterns, together with their own experiences; and analyzing the various solutions to identified problem situations.

The curriculum first focuses on providing the medical information that the well sibling lacks about a brother or sister's illness and treatment that limits communication within the family system, the peer-group system, and between well siblings and health professionals (Spinetta, 1978, 1981; Gogan & Slavin, 1981; Kramer, 1984). It also addresses the problem of the well siblings' anxiety about their own health (Binger, 1978; Cairns, Clark, Stephen, Smith & Lansky, 1979), and the fantasies that somehow the well siblings were responsible for the disease (Binger, 1973; Gogan & Slavin, 1981).

Throughout the curriculum, in order to confront "cognitive confusion," the medical view about causality of the disease and its treatment is reiterated; the well sibling's own "private version" of the disease is elicited; and emphasis is placed on the fact that simultaneity or sequence does not necessarily imply cause (Sourkes, 1980), with explicit statements from health professionals that, "Nothing anyone did, said, or thought was responsible for the disease" (Koch, Herman & Donaldson, 1974).

The focus of the curriculum then shifts from medical information to information about the pattern of emotions that is both normal and acceptable as well siblings cope with the changes in their own lives because a brother or sister has cancer. Shame, embarrassment and concern that their family is different (Cunningham, Betsa & Gross, 1973); anger because of the disruption in the family as a result of the disease (Albin, Binger, Stein, Kushner, Zoger & Mikkelson, 1971); guilt about their own health and unrestricted activities (Kramer, 1984); jealousy and resentment as emotional realignment in the family system occurs due to overprotectiveness by parents of ill siblings (Gogan & Slavin, 1981); and the resentment that can be bi-directional when ill siblings are angry at their brothers and sisters for being well (Kagen-Goodheart, 1977) are all reviewed in a non-judgmental framework.

Patterns of behavior are identified next, when well siblings withdraw from peers, or become more aggressive when defending sick brothers and sisters (Kramer, 1984). Behavior may produce poor school performance (Binger, 1969), or evidence a need for punishment and for attention as the well siblings become more accident-prone (Cairns, Clark, Smith and Lansky, 1979

The curriculum ends on a positive note because the well siblings can grow from the experience (Kramer, 1984). Well siblings help each other to identify situational problems, review the medical information as well as the information on patterns of emotions and patterns of behavior, then analyze the positive and negative solutions to those problem situations.

This course will contribute to the education of children as they acquire the skills to communicate comfortably with their families and with health professionals. They will develop problem-solving skills after learning about cancer as a medical disease, and about cancer as it affects the family. They will come to an understanding of the need to reorganize the family during the various phases of disease. They will develop awareness of the feelings and attitudes of the family, staff, peer group and themselves through increased empathy, further develop their powers of observation, and learn to respond more effectively to their own needs and to the needs of their family. Children will develop positive attitudes about the quality of their own life and the quality of their family life. "Cancer: A Curriculum for Well-siblings of Pediatric Cancer Patients" is but one answer to the need for education to address our concerns about "cancer" in all its aspects.

PURPOSES AND GOALS

The overarching purpose of "Cancer: A Curriculum for Well-siblings of Pediatric Cancer Patients" is to enable children to understand that even though their experience of living in a family with a sibling who has cancer is painful, it also is an experience from which they can grow by learning to deal with it progressively. By viewing cancer as a situational problem, they can better learn to cope with present and future problems. They can find new, better, and more creative solutions than have been found by others in the past. By viewing cancer as a catastrophic illness which creates a situational problem, they can better learn to value the quality of life, to value themselves, and to value other people as they learn to cope. By viewing cancer as a situational problem that affects thinking, feeling, and action, they can better learn how to bring thinking, feeling, and action together to understand the problem and to develop creative solutions.

General Statement of Goals

   I. Conceptual
      A. The sibling will develop an understanding of cancer and its treatment.
      B. The sibling will develop an understanding of the physical and emotional effects of cancer.
  II. Inquiry
      A. The sibling will develop the ability to identify problems and formulate questions to ask adults (family members, hospital staff) about the physical and emotional effects of cancer on family members, including parents, patients, and siblings.
 III. Affective
      A. The sibling will develop a positive self image.
      B. The sibling will develop an understanding of his/her values and increase decision-making skills.
      C. The sibling will develop an awareness of the feelings, attitudes, and behavior in the interaction between self, sibling, and parents as affected by the stress of cancer on family life.
  IV. Skills
      A. The sibling will develop interpersonal skills of communication with family members, hospital staff, and peers, both verbally and non-verbally.

Statement of Objectives

   As a result of study, students will be able to:

(Conceptual)
   1. Understand the vocabulary used when talking about cancer;
   2. Understand that cancer is not contagious, nor is it caused or prevented by thoughts, feelings or actions of siblings;

3. Understand differential cancer treatments such as surgery (amputation), chemotherapy, and radiation therapy;
4. Distinguish between normal cells and runaway cells in cell division;
5. Comprehend how cancer treatment can result in the destruction of cancer cells, but produce temporary side effects that make the patient feel worse.

(Inquiry)

6. Question hospital staff about the physical and emotional effects of cancer and its treatment on their ill sibling;
7. Question hospital staff about their distinct professional roles in caring for an ill sibling;
8. Formulate the questions to ask parents;
9. Formulate the questions to ask ill siblings.

(Affective)

10. Understand the normal feelings that siblings and family members experience when a sibling has cancer (anxiety, fear, anger, resentment, protectiveness, jealousy, isolation, abandonment, rejection, guilt, rivalry, low self-worth, sadness, depression, shame);
11. Understand the losses that siblings and family members experience when a sibling has cancer (loss of attention, loss of time, loss of activities, loss of fun, loss of social functioning, loss of love);
12. Identify the behavioral symptoms that surface as a well sibling tries to cope with feelings that emerge because an ill sibling has cancer (school problems, risk taking, overeating, undereating, accident proneness, television addiction, seclusion, conflicts with family members and/or peers);
13. Identify optimal coping strategies to deal with the pain the well sibling experiences when an ill sibling has cancer;
14. Understand the difficult transition periods when the ill sibling returns home or returns to the hospital;
15. Understand the bi-directionality of the sibling-patient relationship;
16. Understand attitudes about cancer and treatment that foster emotional distance within family systems by identifying those attitudes in specific problem situations.

(Skills)

17. Use problem solving skills to include a peer-as-a-partner in decision making that involves alternatives for optimal coping within a family system affected by cancer;

18. Actively listen to a peer and/or hospital staff person, observe and interpret the verbal and non-verbal messages that produce positive and negative communication;
19. The well sibling will formulate a problem situation and display a creative and adequate solution with regard to being a well sibling in a family caring for an ill sibling with cancer;
20. Critique and evaluate the material used in the course with the sibling's own experience continually throughout the course.

ESSENTIAL COMPONENTS OF THE CURRICULUM

The following outline covers the basic content of the curriculum, but teachers are expected and encouraged to fill out the details.

I. Knowledge of Cancer, Treatment and Effects of Treatment
A. Definition of Cancer
B. Nature of Cancer
  1. Normal cell growth
    a. Cell division
    b. Cell differentiation
    c. Cell regulation
  2. Abnormal cell growth
    a. Cell alteration
    b. Changed rate of multiplication
    c. Lack of control
C. General Types of Childhood Cancer
  1. Leukemia
    a. Bone marrow
    b. White blood cells (fight infection)
      1. Granulocytes
      2. Lymphocytes-lymphoblast
      3. Monocytes
    c. Red blood cells (carry oxygen to tissues)
      1. Hemoglobin
      2. Reticulocytes
    d. Platelets (stops bleeding)
  2. Solid Tumors
D. How Cancer Spreads
  1. Local extension
  2. Metastasis
E. Diagnoses
  1. Blood Tests

    2. Bone marrow aspirations

    3. Biopsy

    4. X-rays

F. What Causes Cancer

    1. Specific cause unknown—predisposing causes

    2. Cancer is not contagious—not caused by a germ

    3. Words, thoughts and single injuries do not cause cancer

    4. Nobody can prevent leukemia

    5. Newest information

G. Cancer Treatment

    1. Surgery

       a. Remove malignant tumors

       b. Amputations—limbs/prothesis

    2. Chemotherapy

       a. Needle intravenous

       b. Drugs

          Temporary Side Effects

          1. Nausea

          2. Mouth sores (hurts to eat hot, cold, spicy food, and hurts to talk)

          3. Hair loss - 2 weeks to 2 months after chomotherapy starts

             - falls out all at once or over period of time

             - same person, but looks different

             - sad

             - wears wig, cap, scarf

          4. Decrease in red blood cells, white blood cells, or platelets

             - tired, pale, or cranky

             - more likely to get infection

             - need to avoid crowded places or people who are sick (chicken pox more serious)

             - bruise or bleed more easily

             - need to stay away from rough play

          5. Mood swings

    3. Radiation therapy (X-ray, radium, radiosotopes)

       a. Aimed at cancerous tumor to damage cells ability to divide

       b. Normal cells close to tumor may also get damaged by radiation, but most cells protected by special lead shield placed over other parts of body

       c. Dye or magic markers used to mark area stays on until treatment is over

       d. Radiation machine is very large, but not unlike X-rays for teeth or

broken bones
   e. Treatment takes a few minutes and is given over period of several
      weeks
   f. Person not radioactive after or during radiation
   g. Treatment does not hurt
      Temporary Side Effects
      1. Tired
      2. Area sore like a bad sunburn
      3. Hair may fall out
      4. Nausea
      5. Headaches
      6. Diarrhea
      7. Sore mouth
II. Affective and Behavioral Responses to Childhood Cancer
A. Cognitive Confusion about Causality of Cancer
   1. Simultaneity or sequence of an intensely emotional and incomprehensible
      set of events is often applied to causality. The well sibling thinks pri-
      vately that words, thoughts and behavior caused the disease (magical
      thinking)
   2. Invisibility or visibility of the disease often contributes to confusion.
   3. Temporary side effects of treatment that makes a sick sibling look and
      feel worse, while it is helping sibling get better, contributes to confusion.
   4. Gaps in information, and lack of knowledge about childhood cancer and
      treatment, compound the confusion.
   5. Feelings of guilt and anxiety are often overwhelming when well siblings
      hold secret thoughts that they caused their brothers or sisters to beome
      sick.
   6. Feelings of fear and anxiety emerge when well siblings think that cancer
      is contagious.
   7. Important to elicit private thought about causality first, then explicitly
      state nothing anyone said, did, or thought caused the disease, or could
      have prevented it. Childhood cancer is not contagious.
B. Family Relationships are Affected by Childhood Cancer.
   1. Well siblings are concerned their families are "different" from other
      families.
   2. Family communication is disrupted. The well siblings are often not at the
      family conferences when diagnosis and treatment regimen is discussed,
      resulting in gaps in information, and hesitation to discuss the ill sibling's
      disease with emotionally distraught family members.
   3. Physical separation occurs when the well sibling cannot easily visit the

hospital, or is "boarded out" at the homes of friends and relatives. Communication is often by telephone.

4. Emotional realignment occurs in family system as mother, father and sick child form a triad to cope with the child's illness. Parents often feel emotionally and physically drained, and well sibling feels "left out."

5. Special privileges and extra attention given to the sick child, by parents who often overprotect that child, produces feelings of sibling rivalry, jealousy, anger, rejection and low self-worth in the well child.

6. Parents become more demanding and less tolerant of well siblings.

7. Adolescents, struggling with issues of dependence/independence often feel they are responsible for taking care of the sick sibling and the family.

8. Social activities are restricted when illness and therapeutic regimen prevent families from doing what they used to do together.

9. Emotional responses of well siblings include guilt, anger, rejection, fear, anxiety, loneliness, sadness, shame, embarrassment, and low self-worth.

10. Behavioral responses of well siblings include school problems, somatic illnesses, and vulnerability to accidents.

C. Bi-directional Sibling Relationships are Affected by Childhood Cancer.

1. Negative aspects

a. Normal jealousy among siblings is heightened because the sick siblings get special attention from parents, are overprotected, while more is demanded of the well sibling.

b. Healthy siblings are angry at sick siblings for disrupting the family, and sick siblings are angry at well siblings for being healthy.

c. Healthy siblings feel guilty because they are healthy and enjoy unrestricted play activities while ill siblings are homebound or hospitalized.

d. Healthy siblings often become overprotective of ill siblings, even when the ill siblings are older, reversing the role relationship.

e. Medication results in lethargy and moodiness, and therepeutic regimen changes the sick siblings' personality and physical appearance, straining sibling relationships.

f. Siblings learning about, or witnessing painful procedures, without understanding them, finds them frightening, confirms threat to sick siblings' lives, and raises anxiety over well siblings' own vulnerability to illness.

2. Positive aspects

a. Healthy and ill siblings empathize with each other, care for each other, and express their love for each other.

b. Siblings mature from the experience, develop inner strength, become more tolerant of others, develop positive attitudes.

c. Well siblings value good health.

d. Siblings make the most of each day.

D. Peer Relationships are Affected by Childhood Cancer.

1. Well siblings become moody, withdrawn, and feel they have no one to talk to who understands what they are going through.

2. Peers and friends withdraw when they do not know what to say, have little knowledge of childhood cancer, and think the well siblings want to be left alone.

3. Peers tease sick siblings because of overweight or loss of hair. Well siblings feel embarrassed, angry, confused, and withdraw or become overprotective.

KEY TERMS

alkylating agents	glass slide	prosthesis
amputation	hematology	RNA
antibiotics	hemoglobin	radiation therapy
antimetabolite	hormone	sarcoma
bacteria	immunology	scalpel
benign	infection	spleen
biopsy	intravenous (IV)	side effects
cancer	leukemia	surgery
carcinogen	lymph node	stoma
carcinoma	lymphoma	thymus gland
chemotherapy	malignant tumor	tumor
DNA	mastectomy	vinca alkaloids
diagnosis	metastasis	virus
drug	molecule	X-rays
endocrinology	oncology	situational problem
enzyme	oxygen	
exfoliative cytology	role	

ORGANIZATION

The well siblings will be divided into two groups (ages 6 through 12, and 13 through 17). They will meet simultaneously, so that families who have children in both groups will have only one trip to make. Three groups of well siblings divided into early childhood, middle childhood, and adolescence, would be more appropriate to meet the differential cognitive, emotional, behavioral and experiential factors involved in each group, but availability of staff will affect the choice. More trusting relationships are developed in a multi-session program, but the program would run for one day because of the risk of attrition.

The learning experiences are organized to take a sequential, topical approach that moves from a knowledge base of cancer, to theory and to practical application of theory. Appropriate learning activities are structured specifically for active children. The learning activities support each other and do represent a progression that begins with an activity to "break the ice." This activity is planned to help well siblings meet, and feel comfortable with each other as peers with similar experiences. Names and telephone numbers will be exchanged during the day with encouragement to set up a network support system of peers.

This activity will be followed by a discussion period about normal cells and cancer cells, using relevant vocabulary, and age-appropriate explanations of the terminology used when discussing cancer. Age-appropriate audio visual material will support the discussion about cell division. The topic of cancer will be divided into the childhood diseases of leukemia and mass tumors; the main treatments for cancer (surgery, chemotherapy, and radiation); and the permanent and temporary side effects that makes the patient feel worse, but can result in the destruction of cancer cells. The subject matter is divided into the main issues about cancer, so children will not be overwhelmed with too much information during a short period of time. The content taught the older group will of course be more sophisticated than the content taught the younger group, and will connect, expand upon, and clarify what is taught in school classrooms. Physicians and nurses, whose education and training supports their knowledge of the disease and treatment, will teach this component of the curriculum. They will be well qualified to ask siblings what they think causes cancer, answer the questions siblings raise, and help siblings to formulate their own questions and answers. This is planned to help clarify any misconceptions children have about the cause of cancer, establish a communication system between medical staff and well siblings, and enable siblings to discuss the information they have learned with parents, ill siblings, and peers. Social workers will also begin to elicit the children's unexpressed fears about causality, so they do not hold on to their own "private versions" while accepting medical explanations. Doctors, nurses, and social workers will teach the children that sequence and simultaneity do not necessarily produce causality. They will elicit emotional concerns about causality, then explicitly state that thoughts and behavior do not cause cancer. Social workers will also carefully help the siblings to connect the intellectual knowledge of the effects of the treatment of cancer with a few of the feelings that emerge, when they discuss hair loss, loss of a limb, or change in body weight. The discussions will enable well siblings to recognize they are not alone, that those same feelings are experienced by other well siblings, and that it is safe to discuss them as normal feelings.

The discussion period will be followed by an activity to enable well siblings to move around the hospital in groups and to clarify the knowledge they gained in the earlier period. The well siblings will be given a choice of a tour of the hospital to see the equipment used to treat cancer. They will have the opportunity to compare cancer cells with healthy cells under a microscope, in order to reinforce their new knowledge of cell division and dispel the cognitive confusion about causality. They will be shown and allowed to handle regular hospital materials (syringes, needles with the tips cut, intravenous tubing and bottles, tongue depressors, stethoscopes, surgical masks and gloves, blood pressure sets, bandages and reflex hammers), and told how the equipment is used to help their brothers and sisters.

After the tour, and lunch, the well siblings will participate in non-competitive games arranged by the recreation therapist, whereby everyone will be a winner. This is a special day for siblings, and special efforts should be made to make them feel good about themselves and each other. A supportive network is encouraged to develop among well siblings.

Following the games, a discussion group will focus on the normal feelings that emerge as well siblings cope with the trauma of cancer in the family. Social workers will encourage and support well siblings to share their experiences, and their feelings. Vignettes will be used to present theoretical problem situations that involve a well sibling in an interaction with his or her environment. The vignettes will include relationships and communication with siblings, parents, friends, peers, neighbors, and schoolmates. Such vignettes are designed to combine the child's experiences, emotions, and behavior with the existing body of knowledge of cancer and its physical, emotional and behavioral effects on the well sibling. They will include behavioral symptoms that evidence adaptive and maladaptive coping mechanisms, positive and negative bi-directionality within the sibling system, emotional realignment and balanced alignment of the family system, closed and open communication patterns and attitudes that foster emotional distance or cohesive relationships, and the value of making the most of each day. The vignettes will be open-ended to allow the well siblings to formulate the problem situations they identify with, and discuss creative and adequate solutions. This is planned to enable the well siblings to develop a sense of mastery over situations that can be overwhelming, make them feel good about themselves as they strengthen adaptive coping skills and effective thinking to solve problems they are experiencing, or that may arise in the future.

The day will end on a social note to enable siblings to unwind, enjoy the relationships they formed during the day, and have fun. Dancing and game playing activities are planned by the recreation therapist.

LEARNING EXPERIENCES

The learning experiences are organized to support each other and to form a natural progression, as described above. Although it is important to follow the order for progression, the program must remain flexible in order to meet the needs of the well siblings. The resource material mentioned in the following list is described more fully on page 112–113.

It is also important for teachers and health professionals to evaluate each well sibling throughout the course. Any sibling exhibiting stressful behavior should be given individual support and attention. Siblings evidencing the need of extra support should be identified, and plans made for follow-up care. Well siblings are vulnerable, and caution should be taken that they feel good about themselves.

1. Students participate in an "ice-breaking" activity to meet and feel comfortable with each other. Further activities should enable a supportive network to develop among well siblings.
2. Students participate in a lecture and discussion about cancer, the treatment of cancer and the effects of treatment.
3. Students develop a unit for descriptive language about the vocabulary specific to cancer by listing words on the blackboard, and analyzing the meaning of those words.
4. Students view the film *From One Cell* (American Cancer Society), discuss, and critique.
5. Students identify who in their family has cancer, what type of cancer, and how it is being treated.
6. Students locate and describe the location of cancer in their brothers or sisters on a large diagram of the body, placed in front of the room. They will use the vocabulary specific to cancer.
7. Students view overhead transparencies, "Cell Structure and Function" (American Cancer Society), and report how that information is useful or not useful when applied to their understanding of cancer in their siblings.
8. Students report on how they think the physical examination of their sisters or brothers detected clues to cancer.
9. Students help each other to formulate the questions to ask health professionals about cancer, the treatment of cancer, and the effects of that treatment.
10. Students identify the different health professions, and the special care each professional group provides for their sick siblings.

11. Students actively listen to the responses from each professional group to clarify the information they are given.
12. Health professionals elicit from the students what the students think caused the cancer in their sick siblings. Responses of simultaneity or unrelated sequences of events that reflect magical thinking will be encouraged.
13. Health professionals will discuss with students how thoughts, actions, and behavior are often thought to cause cancer, but do not. Students' "secret thoughts" about causality are elicited as a basis for discussion. The idea that thoughts, actions and behavior cannot cause or prevent cancer in sick siblings will be repeated throughout the course. Everyday situations involving simultaneity and unrelated sequences of events will be presented and analyzed in order to show they do not necessarily prove causality.
14. Health professionals will discuss with students how and why cancer is not contagious, while reviewing the diseases that are in fact contagious (measles, mumps, colds).
15. Students report in a free discussion with health professionals what misconceptions exist with regard to the cause of cancer.
16. Students identify persons (in the hospital, the family, and the community) to whom they can go to talk about cancer in their family; identify persons they would like to talk to, but cannot; and analyze why it is easier to talk about cancer to some people, but not others.
17. Students are assisted by health professionals to formulate the questions they would like to ask their ill siblings, and the information they would like to share.
18. Students engage in role play, "talking to" sick brothers and sisters, and analyze responses.
19. Students are assisted by health professionals to formulate the questions they would like to ask their parents, and the information they would like to share.
20. Students role-play talking to parents about that information, and analyze the responses.
21. Students discuss how their peers react to the sick siblings and to themselves and identify the problems that surface in the interactions.
22. Students role-play the various interactions between peers/sick siblings, peers/well siblings, sick siblings/peers/well siblings, then critique the responses and consequences, and analyze the solutions.
23. Students are assisted by health professionals to plan what they can teach their peers and their friends about cancer and the effect of cancer.

24. Students discuss and analyze why cancer education is important, and how they are affected by misinformation and a lack of knowledge about childhood cancer in their schools and community.
25. Students conduct a panel discussion on the part that elementary and high school students can play in educating students about cancer.
26. Students take a tour of the hospital to see the equipment used to help sick siblings.
27. Students will view normal cells and cancer cells under a microscope, compare and analyze their differences, and discuss the consequences of the different behaviors of those cells (Baker, 1978).
28. Students will report on a cytological slide after a visit to the laboratory (American Cancer Society, 1975).
29. Students will report on a biopsy as described by a physician or a laboratory technician (American Cancer Society, 1975).
30. Students will discuss, critique, and integrate information about cancer with their experiences of living in a family with a sibling who has cancer.
31. Students will participate in non-competitive games to enable a supportive network to develop among well siblings, and help them feel good about themselves.
32. Students will discuss and analyze why the treatment to destroy cancer cells often makes sick siblings feel and look worse than before the treatment.
33. Younger students will draw a picture (on paper or on the blackboard) showing how sick siblings looked before the illness and after the treatment of the illness (no hair, missing limb, overweight, underweight).
34. Younger students will look into hand mirrors, and share what they notice about their eyes and hair. They will cover their hair and discuss whether or not they would be different inside if they had no hair.
35. Younger students will analyze how sick siblings are different outside, and how they are the same person inside.
36. Students will discuss different feelings (good and bad) they have experienced since their siblings became ill. Health professionals will reassure students those feelings are normal and acceptable, as they list them on a blackboard.
37. Younger students will make "feeling mirrors" to mirror their own moods and emotions and respond to the other students' moods and emotions. They will analyze how other childrens' moods affect their own moods and behavior. (Teachers Guide, American Cancer Society)

38. Students discuss behavioral responses to those feelings, and analyze the good and bad consequences of different behaviors.
39. Younger students will diagram a decision-making chain (he/she felt badly because . . . he/she fought with a friend . . . took dumb chances . . . felt worse). Students will analyze how the process might be changed. (Teacher's Guide, American Cancer Society)
40. Younger students will use the Poster "Special People" (Teacher's Guide, American Cancer Society) to discuss and analyze the various children in the poster. What are they like? Who are their friends? What are their special talents and interests? How do they take care of themselves? How do they feel about themselves? Students will choose one of the children in the poster to think through a story, imagining each child was a well sibling with a sick brother or sister. They will include their character's feelings about themselves as well as the major events in their lives. They will also include the behavior evidenced by each character (riding a bicycle with no hands past a stop sign, eating junk food, watching television, pushing a handicapped child's wheelchair, sulking in a room, riding a skateboard without looking ahead, joining a music group, laughing at someone who looks different).
41. Students will discuss different situations that caused good and bad feelings, resulting in differential behavior (parental overprotectiveness of sick siblings, gaps in family communication, increased responsibility, activities cancelled owing to therapeutic regimen of sick siblings, loss of attention when sick siblings return home or are hospitalized, friends who don't understand).
42. Students will discuss and critically analyze the positive and negative bi-directionality of sibling relationships using examples such as the emotional realignment of family members, the overprotective attitude of parents toward sick siblings and more demanding behavior toward well siblings.
43. Students will write on an index card a problem they experienced involving peers, parents or sick siblings. Three groups will be formed, each to deal with one of the three sets of problems (peers, parents or ill siblings). Each group will take the cards related to that group and create vignettes of problem situations that include the majority of problems written up, identify all the feelings involved, and include several different behaviors to respond to the problems. Each group will present their vignettes to the audience in whichever way they feel comfortable (role playing, acting in a television program, discussion panels). The audience will participate in analyzing

the good and the bad consequences of each of the behaviors, and share their reactions. The actors will tell the audience why they said or did the things in the way they portrayed the scene. The group and audience will come to their own conclusions.

44. Younger students will create one-minute television commercials about themselves to state in a positive way something they did that was terrific, and made them feel good about themselves, or something they plan to do that involves them and their family. (Teacher's Guide, American Cancer Society)

45. Students will write up short "quality of life" statements, including the value of living each day fully, and share those statements with other students.

SUMMARY

A curriculum was developed by the author that would provide children with the cognitive, affective, and behavioral information about the biological, medical, and contextual aspects of cancer, using their past and present experiences, to enable them to cope in a better way with their situational problem of cancer. It is designed to help children to solve problems specific to living with a sibling who has cancer, and also to set the precedent for solving later problems that arise due to separation, loss, or death. Parents are often relieved that their children will learn to cope in a better way with the trauma of having a sibling ill with cancer, which in turn can provide parents with more energy to help ill children fight the disease. Communication between parents and children should be enriched, which will enable the family members to enjoy a better quality of life.

The curriculum is also important in providing health professionals not only with a course to educate children about cancer, but also with a tool to educate themselves about the problems families are facing when the diagnosis is cancer. It will enable health professionals to care for pediatric cancer patients with a greater awareness of the patient as a brother or sister in a familial setting that has become disorganized because of the disease.

It is hoped that "Cancer: A Curriculum for Well-siblings of Pediatric Cancer Patients" will be recognized as a model from which many valuable curricula can be developed to meet the needs of diverse populations in a world affected by cancer.

RESOURCES FOR EDUCATORS

Printed Materials from American Cancer Society
Teaching About Cancer: A Guide to Source Materials and Information, 1975.

Proceedings of the National Conference on the Care of the Child with Cancer, 1978.
When You Have a Student With Cancer, 1980.
American Cancer Society Proceedings of the Third National Conference on Cancer Nursing, 1981.
The Nature of Cancer (Teaching Kit)
Study Guide for the Film, *From One Cell*
Teachers Guide—Grades K-8
Overhead Transparencies from American Cancer Society
"Cell Structure and Function"
"The Nature of Cancer"
Films from American Cancer Society
From One Cell (revised 1978)
Film
Baker, Lynn S. *You and Leukemia—A Day at a Time*. W.B. Saunders Company, Philadelphia, 1978.
National Cancer Institute
Students With Cancer: A Resource for the Educator, 1980.
For Children and Adolescents When Someone in Your Family has Cancer, 1983.
Schweers, E.W., et al. Parents' Handbook on Leukemia. The American Cancer Society, 1977.
Sherman, Mikie. The Leukemic Child. National Institutes of Health, 1982.
Shimkin, Michael B. Science and Cancer. National Institutes of Health, 1980.

REFERENCES

ADAMS-GREENLY, M. AND R.T. MOYNIHAN. 1983. "Helping the Children of Fatally Ill Parents." *American Journal of Orthopsychiatry* 53:219–229.

ALBIN, A.R., C.M. BINGER, R.C. STEIN, J.H. KUSHNER, S. ZOGER, AND C. MIKKELSON. 1971. "A Conference with the Family of a Leukemic Child." *American Journal of Diseases of Children* Vol. 122, October.

BINGER, C.M., A.R. ABLIN, R.C. FUERSTEIN, J.H. KUSHNER, S. ZOGER, AND C. MIKKELSON. 1969. "Childhood Leukemia—Emotional Impact on Patient and Family." *New England Journal of Medicine* 280 (8): 414–418.

BINGER, C. 1973. Childhood Leukemia: Emotional Impact on Siblings. In E.G. Anthony, and C. Koupernik eds. *The Child in His Family: Impact of Disease and Death*. New York: John Wiley and Sons.

CAIRNS, N.U., G.M. CLARK, D. STEPHEN, M.D. SMITH, AND S.B. LANSKY. 1979. "Adaptation of Siblings to Childhood Malignancy." *The Journal of Pediatrics* Vol. 95, September.

CAIN, A., I. FAST, AND M. ERICKSON. 1964. "Children's Disturbed Reactions to the Death of a Sibling." *American Journal Orthopsychiatry* 34.

CUNNINGHAM, C., N. BETSA, AND S. GROSS. 1981. "Sibling Groups: Interaction with Siblings of Oncology Patients." *American Journal Pediatrics, Hematology, Oncology* Summer 3(2): 135–9.

DUBERLEY, J. 1979. The Role of Nursing Staff in Helping the Hospitalised Child. In L. Burton, *Care of the Child Facing Death*. London and Boston: Routledge & Kegan Paul.

GOGAN, J.L. AND L.A. SLAVIN. 1981. Interviews with Brothers and Sisters. In G.P. Koocher, and J.E. O'Malley, *The Damocles Syndrome: Psychosocial Consequences of Surviving Childhood Cancer*. New York: McGraw Hill.

HEFFRON, W.A., K. BOMMELAERE, AND R. MASTERS. 1973. "Group Discussions with the Parents of Leukemic Children." *Pediatrics* 52: 841–840.

KAGEN-GOODHEART, L. 1977. "Re-entry: Living with Childhood Cancer." *American Journal of Orthopsychiatry* 47: 651–658.

KOCH, C.R., J. HERMANN, AND M.H. DONALDSON. 1974. "Supportive Care of the Child with Cancer and His Family." *Seminars in Oncology* 1: 81–86.

KRAMER, R.F. 1984. "Living with Childhood Cancer: Impact on the Healthy Siblings." *Oncology Nursing Forum* Vol II, No. 1, Jan/Feb.

LANSKY, S.B. AND J.T. LOWMAN. 1974. "Childhood Malignancy: A Comprehensive Approach." *The Journal of the Kansas Medical Society* March 75(3): 91–94.

MCCOLLUM, A.T. 1974. Counselling the Grieving Parent. In L. Burton, *Care of the Child Facing Death.* London and Boston: Routledge & Kegan Paul.

SOURKES, B. 1980. Siblings of the Pediatric Cancer Patient. In *Psychological Aspects of Childhood Cancer.* Springfield: Charles C. Thomas.

SOURKES, B. 1977. "Facilitating Family Coping with Childhood Cancer." *Journal of Pediatric Psychology* 2:34–45.

SPINETTA, J.J. 1978. Communication Patterns in Families Dealing with Life-Threatening Illness. In O.J.Z. Sahler, *The Child and Death.* St. Louis: C.V. Mosby Company.

SPINETTA, J.J. 1981. The Sibling of the Child with Cancer. In J.J. Spinetta, and Deasy-Spinetta, *Living with Childhood Cancer.* St. Louis: C.V. Mosby Company.

12

Cancer and the Family: Experiences of Children and Adolescents

Edythe S. Ellison, RN, PhD

The maintenance of the integrity of the family unit as a potential source of support for persons with cancer has long been espoused by health care professionals. Nevertheless, there is an appalling lack of reliable information on the day-to-day experiences and problems of families in which a member has cancer. Furthermore, the studies that have been done suffer from a number of limitations. Case studies and analytical papers with limited practical implications, such as those by Parkes (1975) and Weisman and Worden (1976), predominate in the literature. Few studies have documented information from more than one family member, usually the husband (Chekryn 1984; Lieber et al. 1976; Vachon et al. 1977; Wellisch, Jamison, and Pasnau 1978). Studies that consider children tend to focus on the adult children of older patients (Germino 1984).

Another limitation of family-based studies of cancer is that they tend to focus on the early diagnosis or the late stages of the disease (Gotay 1984; Grobe, Ahmann, and Ilstrup 1982). Thus little information is available to guide the development of services to families during the time in which the disease may be in remission. In addition, because studies of families with cancer have been limited by single-group designs, little is known about the differences that may exist according to the specific diagnosis.

Moreover, primarily negative effects have been reported from small samples and case studies. The possibility that children can cope with or even benefit from experiences surrounding a parent's illness has not been suggested. This is striking in light of the reported natural resiliency and "self-righting" qualities of children that have been observed under a variety of stressors (Sameroff and Chandler 1975). One question, then, is, How do families assist children to cope with the stresses of a parent's chronic illness, particularly one like breast cancer, so their resiliency and self-righting qualities become actualized? Other pertinent questions that have not been dealt with are these: How do families inform children of a parent's illness? How do they communicate with children after the initial crisis is over? and What perceptions of the illness do the children have?

RESEARCH DESIGN AND PURPOSES

The data presented here are part of a larger research effort that was designed to take into account many of the aforementioned limitations and issues. The Family Impact Study (Lewis, Woods, and Ellison 1986) is a three-year federally funded research project concerned with the impact of a mother's chronic illness on the family. Utilizing a three-group comparison design, the researchers studied 129 families with a total of 171 children: 55 in which the mothers had breast cancer, 32 in which the mother had diabetes, and 42 in which the mother had fibrocystic breast disease. Data were collected over an 18-month period. Families were interviewed at home on three to five occasions using a combination of self-administered questionnaires, interviews with the whole family, and interviews with individual family members. The study consisted of eight broad themes: the perceived demands of the illness, the quality of the marital relationship, the social support available to the family, the family's ability to cope, the quality of the parent–child relationship, the psychosocial functioning of parents and children, and the functioning and health of the entire family.

Another part of the study systematically documented the child's perceptions of the mother's illness. The data were collected within a structured interview, the Child's Perception of Mother's Illness, designed specifically for the study (Ellison 1983). (See Figure-1 for the interview questions.) The first group of questions was concerned with who informed the child about the mother's illness, when the child was informed, what the child recalled being told about the illness, and what he or she thought or felt at the time. The child was then asked what he or she knew about the mother's health. A subsequent group of questions assessed what changes may have occurred in the child's life since the mother's illness and how the child felt about them. A final question asked the child to share three wishes with the interviewer. The children were encouraged to express themselves as much as they felt comfortable. The data were gathered and analyzed with the intent of having the subjects provide their own construction and experience of being informed about and living with their mothers' cancer. Validity rested in the subjects' reports of their experiences as they evaluate them and as they appeared to the subjects at the time of the interview.

The mothers in the study were patients with nonmetastatic breast disease who were diagnosed by a physician as being in remission on their entrance in the study. They were mostly educated middle-class and upper-middle class caucasian women with one or more school-aged children living at home.

DATA ANALYSIS AND RESULTS

Data from the interviews were subjected to two methods of analysis. First, all data from the three diagnostic groups (breast cancer, diabetes, and fibrocystic breast disease) were subjected to a content analysis that yielded 128 categories of responses. The number of responses within the 128 categories ranged from one to 39, with an average of 11 responses per child. Using theoretical coding, 10 theoretically consistent categories (or composite categories) emerged from the original 128. Intercoder reliability was assessed and ranged from .88 to .96.

The first three composite categories are concerned with the extent to which the child was informed about the mother's illness. The *Informed* category includes seven responses by which the child acknowledged being informed about the mother's illness. The second category, *Lack of Information,* consists of six responses by which the child acknowledged a lack of information or expressed dissatisfaction with the information provided. *Facts,* the third composite category, is comprised of 14 types of factual information the child presented about the mother's illness, that is , information pertaining to the diagnosis, treatment, or effects of treatments.

Three additional composite categories represent the child's affective responses to the mother's illness. The *Reassurance* composite category (five items) refers to the child's report of having been reassured by the mother, father, or both and expressions of positive expectations for the mother's health. A category of *Fear, Questions, Concerns* consists of six responses in which the child identified specific or generalized fears, questions, and concerns related to the mother's health. Finally, *Emotional Response* involved the child's reports of intense feelings in response to the mother's diagnosis (eight items).

Two composite categories were concerned with the child's identification of changes (seven each) in individual family members or in the family unit. *Life Change—Positive* consists of changes to which the child reported a positive response and *Life Change—Negative* consists of those to which the child reported a negative response. *Heredity or Vulnerability* is a composite of nine responses by which the child expressed concern regarding his or her vulnerability to or inheritance of the mother's illness. The final category, *Parental Death,* is comprised of five expressions of the child's fear of the mother dying.

Differences in the child's perceptions according to the mother's diagnosis were examined by first calculating means and then comparing them by an analysis of variance. As was previously reported (Ellison, Houck, and Wallace 1985), significant differences among the diagnostic groups were found for five of the ten categories. Children in families in which the mother had breast cancer scored significantly higher than did children in the other two groups in the composite categories of being *Informed,* expressions of *Reassurance,* degree of *Emotional Response,* and *Fears, Questions, and Concerns.* In addition, children in families in which the mother had cancer or diabetes reported significantly more *Facts* than those of families in which the mother had fibrocystic breast disease.

Consequently, it appears that although children of mothers with cancer seem to experience greater emotional intensity when informed of the diagnosis and greater levels of fear and concern, they also report receiving more information and reassurance from their parents to assist them in dealing with their emotions and fears. Thus, we have some preliminary evidence that differences may exist in the demands and intensity of emotional responses associated with a diagnosis of cancer as opposed to diabetes and fibrocystic breast disease. However, the results concerning the degree of reassurance provided suggest that serious consideration be given to expanding the present models that universally predict deleterious effects as a result of cancer in the family to ones that include possibilities for successful coping and perhaps psychological growth, as well.

The second method of analyzing the children's interviews was to subject the data to a qualitative content analysis on a case-by-case basis grouped according to the mother's diagnosis, and the child's age (7–12 years and 13–19 years). All the data from the interviews with the young children and adolescents were first examined independently by two of the investigators. Using an open coding system, the investigators generated similar sets of response categories. The theoretical framework that guided the selective coding was a focus on describing the dimensions and properties of the psychosocial milieu of the illness. The investigators then discussed their separate categories of responses and collaborated on a set of categories that accounted for all the relevant aspects of the child's experiences with the mother's illness. This process resulted in the inclusion of a greater number of statements in relevant categories, reaching the point of saturation where the vast majority of the data were accounted for. The results of this analysis of the data from 84 children whose mothers had cancer, 30 aged 7–12 and 54 aged 13–19 are presented next.

Young Children

Of the 30 children under age 12 whose mothers had breast cancer, two children answered no to the question, "Has either your Mom or Dad talked to you about your Mom's health?" Three children answered,"I can't remember."

The remaining 25 children were able to relate the experience of being told about their mother's illness in specific ways. Often the experience of being told was marked by time ("in 1983," "two years ago," "when I was 3") or the circumstances surrounding the diagnosis and treatment ("when she was in the hospital," "while we were waiting for her to come back from surgery"). Sixteen of the 25 children reported they had been told explicitly that their mother had cancer, and many of them specifically mentioned breast cancer.

The children openly discussed their feelings on being told that their mother had cancer. Three children reported they felt sad, and one child said she felt sorry for her mother. Six of the children expressed their lack of complete understanding about what was going on at the time of their mothers' diagnosis and treatment ("I didn't know what was wrong, I didn't quite understand," "I didn't know what to expect," " I didn't know what was going to happen; I thought they were going to shoot laser beams into her").

Thirteen of the 30 young children mentioned feeling scared or worried when told about the cancer. ("I was afraid to see her; I thought she might be different" or "I thought I wouldn't see her again"). One girl remarked, "I was a little angry that it happened to her." And four children, two boys and two girls, related feeling a lack of concern or feeling confident that everything would be all right.

In the first interview, 11 children reported no changes in their lives as a result of their mother's diagnosis of breast cancer. Three children reported subtle changes in their mother ("she wears her hair differently," "she has to take it easier"), and six children reported having more responsibility or more housework because of their mother's illness.

Changes in family life that were mentioned included getting more rest (one child), eating better food (one child), and decreased time with the mother or decreased joint activities with the mother (four children). One 11-year-old boy reported becoming closer to his mother because of the diagnosis.

More explicit information emerged in the second through fifth interviews in response to questions regarding their current information about the mother's illness—what they knew or how they felt. With few exceptions, these young children reflected their mother's remission status by remarking that she was doing fine.

The children also offered additional information that was not entirely positive. Five children remarked on their mother's smoking habits and her lung trouble.

A few children mentioned long-term changes in their lives resulting from their mother's cancer. Two children mentioned thankfulness that it was over and increased appreciation of the mother and two others noted increased time spent together. Three children mentioned having to help more (or feeling that they ought to) as semipermanent changes. Finally, one child stated, "She just yells at us more than she used to."

Gender differences were not apparent in the data from these interviews. It is only with the adolescent children (17 boys and 37 girls) that differences according to gender began to emerge.

Older Children

Most of the adolescents could accurately describe their experiences of being told about their mother's illness. They could relate the occasion in time ("about a year and three months ago," "when I was in my junior year," or "four years ago") or circumstances surrounding the treatment or diagnosis ("The last day of school, Mom came home from her physical"; "When she first found out it was cancer, there was a family discussion"; or " She told me before she went in for surgery"). However, three teenagers also spoke of not being told enough. They said, "After she knew she had the illness, they waited for a better diagnosis before they told me." "I didn't know for a while. I think they knew for about a week." "They *told* me, but not enough. I remember how disgusted I was when I found out she had a full mastectomy. I understood what was happening, so they should have been honest with me." Only one child (a 16-year-old boy) reported not being told at all.

The majority of the adolescents reported having negative feelings when they were informed of their mother's illness. Three reported feeling sad or "real emotional," five stated they were shocked, and another three said they felt confused or angry. By far, the most common feeling was fear, reported by 12 children; 10 children specifically mentioned the fear that she would die from the cancer.

Four of the 37 girls reported they had reflected on their previous experiences with cancer; one girl linked her maternal grandmother's cancer with her mother's cancer and felt concern for herself ("I felt oops, I'm next").

When asked to reflect on the changes that occurred in their lives because of their mothers' diagnosis 11 adolescents commented on their mother's symptoms or her responses: lack of energy, being sick a lot, trouble eating, being short tempered.

Increased knowledge and awareness of the disease process was mentioned by 10 girls (but only one boy), and the hereditary nature of breast cancer seemed to be uppermost in many of these girls' minds. Indications that normalization had resulted ("I tried to go live as normally as possible") was mentioned by five boys but only one girl. Seven girls but no boys mentioned an increased appreciation of their mothers. In addition, two girls mentioned that the cancer had brought the family closer together.

Twenty-eight of the 37 older girls were able to verbalize that they knew their mother was currently "OK," and some used the phrase "in remission." In the few cases in which metastases had occurred while the study was in progress, the children indicated that they had been informed and expressed appropriate feelings of worry, fear, and concern.

One of the most frequently mentioned changes had to do with taking more responsibility for the day-to-day management of the house. Here, too, there were apparent differences according to sex, with 11 girls (about a third) but only two boys mentioning this change.

Discussion

An analysis of the interview data indicated that although the diagnosis of breast cancer is associated with fear, sadness, and concern, there were no indications that the children were experiencing serious psychological problems. On other indicators, such as self-esteem measures and overall adjustment scales, all the children's scores fell within the normal ranges (Lewis, Woods, and Ellison 1986).

However, there were indications that the parents needed information on how to assist their children to cope with the stressor of the mother's cancer. Children of all ages indicated a need for clear, concise, developmentally appropriate information about the nature of the disease, its treatment, and issues of contagion and heredity. In addition, differences in responses and behavior according to gender seemed to appear in adolescence, with the girls taking on greater responsibility for household chores and boys demonstrating a tendency to distance themselves and "normalize." This last result is striking, given the prevalence of females among adult children who are caretakers of sick elderly parents.

Table-1 summarizes the principal results of the interview data and presents implications for the design and delivery of health care services to families, and for the design of curricula.

TABLE-1.

Results of the Study and Implications for the
Development of Services and Curricula

Interview Data	Health Care Services	Curricula
Young Children		
Lack accurate information and complete understanding of breast cancer or its treatment.	Family-based treatment protocols must be developed that include assessment of the young child's understanding of the disease, its progress, and its treatment.	Theories and models of child development (psychosocial and cognitive) need to be included.
	Developmentally appropriate materials that present accurate information about cancer and its treatment need to be developed.	Experience in adapting information to be consistent with the variety of levels of cognitive and psychosocial development should be provided.
	Children need direct support services to assist them in integrating thoughts and feelings and communicating them to their parents.	The acquisition of information and skills in interviewing and communicating with children needs to be integrated.
Emotional responses: fear, anger, sadness.	Assessment protocols need to be developed that examine the impact on the child's ongoing development: eating, sleeping, school behavior.	Principles of psychosocial and physical assessment and experiences in their application need to be included.
	Family-support protocols need to be designed to help parents support their children, including information about expected behaviors.	Experiences in family therapy with families with young children need to be included.
	Child-support protocols, including both individual and group therapy models, need to be developed.	Theories and models of individual and group therapy with young children are needed, as well as supervised clinical experiences.
Adolescents		
Incomplete and inaccurate information about breast cancer and its treatment.	Materials presenting information on cancer and its treatment that are consistent with the cognitive development and particular	Information on psychosocial development in adolescence should be included.

concerns of adolescents need to be developed. They must include information on heredity and prevention. Extend the focus of the delivery of services to many levels: individual adolescents, parents, families, and schools.

Experience in adapting information on cancer and its treatment to an adolescent audience should be provided. Information and skill acquisition in interviewing and communicating with children needs to be integrated. Experience in providing services to families as well as community groups (schools) needs to be included.

Emotional responses: fear, anger, sadness.

Family-based treatment protocols must be developed and delivered. Programs should include an assessment of the degree of emotional distress in the adolescent and the effect on psychosocial adjustment and development. Assessment should take account of gender-related differences.

Need to include material related to the developmental tasks of adolescents and the expected and normal range of behavior in response to stress. Psychosocial assessment of adolescents: models and clinical experience. Individual, family, and group therapy (models and clinical experiences) need to be included. The design and delivery of support services to parents and teachers of adolescents should be included.

Figure-1. Child's Perception of Mother's Illness

Introduction
Now I'd like to ask you a few questions regarding what you know about your Mom's health and illness.
1. Has either your Mom or Dad talked to you about your Mom's health?
   When?
   What did they say?
   What did you think (feel) at the time?
2. What do you know about your Mom's health?
3. Can you tell me if there have been any changes in your life (at home) since your Mom and Dad told you about (use words of child to describe Mom's health)?
   What are they?
   What do you think about these changes?

REFERENCES

CHEKRYN, J. 1984. "Cancer Recurrence: Personal Meaning, Communication, and Marital Adjustment." *Cancer Nursing* 7:491–498.

ELLISON, E. S. 1983. "Child's Perception of Mother's Illness." Unpublished interview protocol.

ELLISON, E. S., G. HOUCK, AND K. WALLACE. 1985. " Experiences of Children and Adolescents with Mother's Chronic Illness." Paper presented at the Western Council Higher Education in Nursing Annual Meeting, Seattle, WA.

GERMINO, B. 1984. "Family Members' Concerns After Cancer Diagnosis." Unpublished doctoral dissertation, University of Washington, Seattle.

GOTAY, C. 1984. "The Experience of Cancer during Early and Advanced Stages: The Views of Patients and Their Mates." *Social Science and Medicine* 18:605–613.

GROBE, M. E., D. L. AHMANN, AND D. M. ILSTRUP. 1982. "Needs Assessment for Advanced Cancer Patients and Their Families." *Oncology Nursing Forum* 9:26–30.

LEWIS, F. M., N. F. WOODS, AND E. D. ELLISON. 1986. *Family Impact Study: Cancer and the Family. Final Report.* Seattle: University of Washington School of Nursing.

LIEBER, L., M. M. PLUMB, M. L. GERSTENZANG, AND J. HOLLAND. 1976. "The Communication of Affection between Cancer Patients and Their Spouses." *Psychosomatic Medicine* 38:379–389.

PARKES, C. M. 1975. "The Emotional Impact of Cancer on Patients and Their Families." *Journal of Laryngology and Otolaryngology* 89:1272–1279.

SAMEROFF, A., AND M. CHANDLER. 1975. "Reproductive Risk and Continuum of Caretaking Causality." In D. Horowitz, ed. *Review of Child Development Research*, vol. 4. Chicago: University of Chicago Press, pp. 187–244.

VACHON, M. L. S., K. FREEDMAN, A. FORMO, J. ROGERS, W. A. L. LYALL, AND S. J. J. FREEMAN. 1977. "The Final Illness in Cancer: The Widows' Perspective." *Canadian Medical Association Journal* 117:1151–1154.

WEISMAN, A. D. AND J. W. WORDEN. 1976. "The Existential Plight in Cancer: Significance of the First 100 Days." *International Journal of Psychiatry in Medicine* 7:1–15.

WELLISCH, D. K., K. R. JAMISON, AND R. O. PASNAU. 1978. "Psychosocial Aspects of Mastectomy II: The Man's Perspective." *American Journal of Psychiatry* 135:543–546.

13

Breast Cancer: Living with Uncertainty

Susan B. Westlake, RN, MS
Florence E. Selder, RN, PhD

Breast cancer is the most common malignancy in women in the United States, accounting for 28 percent of all cancers and 18 percent of cancer deaths; one out of 10 women is expected to develop breast cancer in her lifetime (American Cancer Society [ACS] 1988). The majority of women diagnosed with malignant breast disease undergo a modified radical mastectomy, which remains the most common initial treatment approach and the primary mode of therapy (Kinne 1984; Nichols 1982). This procedure, involving removal of the breast and the adjacent axillary lymph nodes, achieves local surgical control of the disease and allows for pathologic staging of the disease, necessary to determine the need for adjunctive treatment (Haskell, Giuliano, Thompson, and Zarem 1985).

Prognosis for the woman with breast cancer is related primarily to the extent of disease at initial diagnosis. The five-year survival rate for women with localized breast cancer has risen from 78 percent in the 1940s to 90 percent today; if the cancer has spread beyond the breast, the rate is reduced to 60 percent (ACS 1988). While the prognosis has improved generally, there is no guarantee that any specific individual woman will find herself among the survivors at a given point in time.

Given the incidence of this disease and the predominant treatment approach, a significant number of women are faced with the diagnosis of a potentially life-threatening disease, disfiguring surgery, and the reality of an uncertain future. At the very least, the experience of breast cancer and its treatment must be viewed as a critical event in a woman's life.

There is a substantial body of literature dealing with the subject of women and breast cancer. In terms of its psychological and social impact, breast cancer has been studied more extensively than any other tumor site (Holland and Mastrovito 1980). Research efforts have been directed toward describing and measuring various aspects of the impact and have included the following major psychosocial correlate study variables: (1) emotional affect state (Ervin 1973; Krouse and Krouse 1982; Maguire 1976; Morris, Greer, and White 1977; Quint 1963; Woods and Earp 1978; Worden and Wiseman 1977); (2) body image and sexuality (Krouse and Krouse 1982; Maguire 1976; Polivy 1977; Quint 1963; Sanger and Reznikoff 1981; Taylor et al. 1985; Woods and Earp 1978); (3) social support (Bullough 1981; Hughes 1982; Jamison, Wellisch, and Pasnau 1978; Peters-Golden 1982; Quint 1963; Woods and Earp 1978); and (4) fear of recurrence (Northouse 1981; Peters-Golden 1982; Quint 1963). Despite the large body of literature that exists, it is difficult to identify any consistent description of women's experiences for, as Meyerowitz (1980) noted, "the findings in the field have been disorganized, disjointed, confusing, and inconclusive" (p. 126).

The purpose of this chapter is (1) to discuss women's responses to the experience of breast cancer and mastectomy, as reported in in-depth, personal interviews (Westlake 1985) and (2) to enhance understanding of these responses by examining them within the framework of *life transition theory* (Selder, as Schmitt 1982). According to this theory, which is grounded in the investigation of personal responses to various events, a life transition is viewed as a passage that follows a critical event disruptive to an existing, personal reality. A life transition bridges the existing reality with an emerging reality. The major characteristic of a life transition is uncertainty. The task of a person in a life transition is to integrate the disrupting event so that it has meaning for the individual experiencing it. During the transition there is an emphasis on regaining one's intactness. Closure of a life transition occurs when the critical event no longer has primary or centrality in the individual's life, and when the sense of self is re-established.

Within this framework, the experience of breast cancer and mastectomy is viewed as a critical event that disrupts a woman's personal reality and threatens her integrity, creating considerable uncertainty. Essential notions she holds about herself (e.g., as healthy and intact) are jeopardized. In the following discussion, responses of women to this event will be examined. Sources of uncertainty in the experience will be identified, as will processes that served to reduce the uncertainty.

The responses to be discussed were drawn from in-depth, tape recorded, open-ended interviews conducted with 11 women who were asked to tell the story of their experience since suspecting or learning they had breast cancer. The women were encouraged to speak freely and openly in their own words of their thoughts, feelings, and responses. An interview guide was used to elicit the chronological unfolding of each woman's story to the present time and to explore her expectations for the future.

The interview tapes were transcribed verbatim and were coded independently by two persons. The data were analyzed in terms of (1) discrete illness and treatment events, (2) the major psychosocial correlates of the experience identified in the literature, and (3) life transition theory processes.

The nonrandomized sample consisted of 11 women, aged 33 to 68 years, who had undergone mastectomy surgery for treatment of primary breast cancer between 9 months and 16 years prior to their participation in the study (Mean: 4.7 years). Participation was limited to women who reported no spread of disease beyond the adjacent axillary lymph node area at the time of, or since, their mastectomy and who currently were not receiving medical treatment for their condition. The goal was to include women who viewed themselves as "cured" in order to explore how they had integrated the cancer experience in their lives.

UNCERTAINTY

Uncertainty is a major characteristic of the life transition experienced by women following the diagnosis of breast cancer. The initial suspicion or detection of a possible malignant condition of the breast is the first awareness a woman has that her personal reality might be changing. Essential notions that she has about her personal health or body integrity are challenged. Further, she becomes aware of the irrevocability and irreversibility of the changed reality very swiftly and dramatically through the confirmation of the breast malignancy and subsequent removal of the breast.

As women move through the illness and treatment experience, they encounter other sources of uncertainty. These include: (1) the treatment decision, (2) the postoperative experience, (3) adjuvant treatment, (4) physical integrity, and (5) the fear of recurrence. These specific sources of uncertainty are summarized in the following discussion of how the uncertainty is reduced.

PROCESSES TO REDUCE UNCERTAINTY

In life transition theory, it is postulated that people seek information to reduce their uncertainty. However, among the women interviewed, only a few sought additional information to reduce their uncertainty. At the time of the diagnosis, the women felt a sense of urgency, that they didn't have time to gather additional information. Further, they reported a primary reliance upon the treatment recommendation of the physician. For example, one woman shared:

And he [the doctor] wanted to schedule surgery, a mastectomy, a modified mastectomy. I could get a second opinion and, uh, but uh, I felt such an urgency, uh, you know, you feel like—get that thing

> out of me. You don't feel you have time. . . . and I felt that if I did
> confer with a doctor who was opposed to the surgery—what do I
> know? I'm just an uneducated person in that area.

Sources of uncertainty reported in the postoperative experience revolved
mainly around the appearance of the breast area and possible disability of the
arm on the affected side. Women who had the opportunity to see and speak
with other women who had had a mastectomy found it helpful. The women
endorsed programs such as the ACS Reach to Recovery program or some kind
of regularly conducted peer support groups. Peer support was viewed as an
example of reducing the uncertainty through comparative testing. This process
reduces uncertainty by the comparison of oneself with others in similar
circumstances. The words of one woman illustrate comparison testing:

> I wondered—how in God's name—how am I going to look?
> . . . . and I'll tell you, women who are laying in the hospital, and
> what have you, I think it's so very important to see somebody come
> in and move their arm and say "Hi, how are you and I'm able to
> do this"—because you really don't think at that point that you can—
> "Will I ever?" or "How am I going to look?"

The provision of social support from spouse, family, and friends was also an
important component in relieving the women's uncertainty about whether they
would be accepted and loved postmastectomy. The demonstration of support
and affection was seen as reaffirming the women's sense of personal value and
positive regard by others.

In the extended postoperative period, no discrete sources of uncertainty
relating specifically to personal skills or attributes were identified in the data.
The women resumed their preoperative level of activities and functions within
a relatively short time. The successful engagement of the women in these
activities was viewed as evidence of the processes of structuring for certainty
through competency testing and normalization. Competency testing involves
determining the presence of a personally valued attribute or skill claimed in the
pre-event reality, such as the ability to manage responsibilities related to home
and employment. Normalization refers to engaging in behaviors that mirror the
standards established by the core society of which one is a member.
Demonstrating competence and engaging in behaviors of healthy, "normal"
women served to reduce the general uncertainty related to the changed reality.

For those women who received adjuvant treatment with chemotherapy or
radiation therapy, sources of uncertainty were identified in relation to the side-
effects of those treatments. The women dealt with this uncertainty primarily

through management strategies of pacing and scheduling activities. Ability to predict the occurrence and duration of side-effects appeared to reduce the uncertainty and allowed subjects to manage their lives accordingly.

Concerns related to body image, physical integrity, sexuality, and appearance were a major source of uncertainty. This uncertainty arose from discovering and adjusting to the complexities associated with living with a mastectomy. The women engaged in a number of processes that reduced the uncertain nature of their life transition, including that of normalization with regard to their physical appearance. All of the women expressed a desire to feel attractive and to appear as normal, breasted women. They attempted to normalize their appearance through the use of a prosthesis and various styles of clothing. One woman commented:

> Now, when I walk around with a slip on, you can't even tell. See,
> I'm very particular now. See, some women might not want to, but
> I like wearing sweaters. No one would ever know in my dance
> class, when I wear tight things or whatever, jump around and all.

Two additional processes that reduced uncertainty were the identification of missed options and the minimization of missed options. Identifying missed options involves the awareness of behaviors or experiences no longer available to the person as a result of the disruptive event. Minimizing missed options involves reducing or mitigating the loss of a pre-event behavior or experience through a process of redefinition, reevaluation, substitution, or avoidance. As one woman shared:

> I had a lot of sundresses that I loved, and forget it. That's one of
> the things I felt bad about, I mean, but, you know, that just—and
> then you say "Hey, I'm still here, so what difference does it make?"
> But that, that's how it is.

This woman was able to minimize the loss of a valued style of clothing that she enjoyed prior to her surgery. For her and many other women, former options no longer available gradually became inconsequential in the face of other issues, such as recurrence of the disease and personal survival.

Fear of disease recurrence was a major source of uncertainty for the women postmastectomy. The recognition of trigger events, described as occurrences that precipitate awareness of the altered reality, was particularly apparent as the women spoke of their concerns about the possibility of disease recurrence.

The first type of trigger event was irrevocability, described as the awareness of the permanence or the irreversibility of the changed reality. As discussed earlier, surgical removal of the breast established this permanent alteration swiftly and dramatically. On the other hand, acknowledgment that one must cope with continuing uncertainty regarding the future, and the possibility of disease recurrence, occurs over time for the person with a malignancy diagnosis. The comments of one woman illustrate this:

> At the end of two years I said to the doctor "Oh, you know, I'm glad I passed the two-year mark." And he must have been having a really bad day. He said "What's so good about that? Why not three? Why not four? Why not five?" Right then it was like, hey, I'm never going to be able to feel good about this. It could always, and I thought, oh boy, will it never end?

The second type of trigger event the women reported in acknowledging awareness of their continuing precarious position was reactivation, described as the awareness of thoughts, feelings, and sensations that occurred earlier in the experience. An example of this is the subject who reported her fears were reactivated at the time of periodic medical check-ups:

> Every time I have to go for a check-up, you always get afraid that they might find something, because the fear is still there and it surfaces at this time of examination. It's probably less now, but I keep expecting I'm not going to feel that way, because I don't feel that way on a day-to-day basis. It always surprises me that I do feel this way. I get real irritable, real crabby, and then I realize what's happening. At first it isn't conscious.

Women dealt with the uncertainty related to disease recurrence primarily though tapping spiritual supports, as well as by distracting themselves from focusing on this concern. There was nothing that the women could do to completely relieve this source of uncertainty, which became a permanent companion of their experience. The fact that these 11 women were willing to discuss, in depth, their personal experience and risk resurfacing and reactivating this uncertainty is acknowledged as a personal act of courage and a gift of themselves.

An interesting finding in the study was the unanimous report of the positive impact of the breast cancer experience. All of the women spoke about somehow being changed by the experience. They reported a revaluing of their lives and a reprioritization of their expenditure of personal time and energy, as illustrated in these comments:

> I'm still the same person, but I've grown through the experience. I look at it as a very positive experience and I think I'm better for it . . . this has been a very growing experience in our lives, what we've been through. Because it makes you really examine what life is really about, what's really important, and what you really want to do.

> The whole touch of cancer makes you look at your life and what you are involved in, and priorities, and taking one day at a time. And people became more precious to me, things less precious; house cleaning, dusting—less important. I think just being, just the fact that I don't have to do, but just to be. I came to accept life was very precious, and thankful to be, just to be. So my time with people, sharing time, with less emphasis on doing, and more thankful for being alive.

This report of the positive impact of the experience is possibly related to the uncertainty reducing process of minimizing missed options. It may also be that the cancer experience confronts a commonly held human superstition that one is immortal. That is, while one knows on a rational level that this is not so, in daily experience one lives as if it were. The diagnosis of a malignant disease clearly and abruptly brings a person face-to-face with the reality of personal mortality. In this sense, the personally held notion of immortality may be viewed as an option that is lost with the diagnosis of malignancy.

It is suggested that the painful, acute awareness or acknowledgment that one's life is limited triggers an introspective inquiry into the meaning of life and the human experience. Such an inquiry also reaffirms that all that really can be known with any certainty is the here and now, and hence the women's shift in reporting living in the present and valuing the here and now. The missed option (i.e., the superstition regarding personal immortality) is redefined as an opportunity to engage more completely in the nature, essence, and experience of being fully human.

An alternative interpretation also is postulated with regard to these revaluing and "presencing" phenomena. The structuring of a new, personally meaningful reality following a disruptive event may involve more than re-establishing or reaffirming one's sense of self as it was known in the previous reality. Perhaps a life transition initiated by awareness of a major change or shift in personal reality carries with it the opportunity for personal enhancement (i.e., growth, creation, or fuller development), an opportunity that would not have been available in the absence of the disruptive event or changed reality. Additionally, these phenomena appear to demonstrate the need to make sense of and find meaning in human experience and one's life, in the face of a disruptive, critical event. As such, they appear to be crucial in allowing one to move through the life transition and integrate the experience within one's life, so that wholeness or personal integrity is maintained and possibly enhanced.

Awareness and understanding of the sources of uncertainty and of the processes that reduce uncertainty may assist health professionals in supporting women who experience the critical disrupting event of breast cancer and mastectomy. Life transition theory provides a valuable framework for this endeavor.

REFERENCES

AMERICAN CANCER SOCIETY. 1988. *Cancer Facts and Figures - 1988.* New York: American Cancer Society.

BULLOUGH, B. 1981. "Nurses as Teachers and Support Persons for Breast Cancer Patients." *Cancer Nursing* 4:221–225.

ERVIN, C. V. 1973. "Psychological Adjustment to Mastectomy." *Medical Aspects of Human Sexuality* 7(2):42–61.

HASKELL, C. M., A. E. GULIANO, R. W. THOMPSON, AND H. A. ZAREM. 1985. "Breast Cancer." In C. M. Haskell, ed. *Cancer Treatment.* Second Edition. Philadelphia: W. B. Saunders, pp. 137–180.

HOLLAND, J. C. AND R. MASTROVITO. 1980. "Psychological Adaptation to Breast Cancer." *Cancer* 46 (Suppl.):1045–1052.

HUGHES, J. 1982. "Emotional Reactions to the Diagnosis and Treatment of Breast Cancer." *Journal of Psychiatric Research* 25:277–283.

JAMISON, K. R., D. K. WELLISCH, AND R. O. PASNAU. 1978. Psychological Aspects of Mastectomy: I. The Woman's Perspective. *American Journal of Psychiatry* 135:432–436.

KINNE, D. W. 1984. "Surgical Management of Clinically Early Breast Cancer." *Cancer* 53(Suppl.):685–690.

KROUSE, H. J. AND J. H. KROUSE. 1982. "Cancer as Crisis: The Critical Elements of Adjustment." *Nursing Research* 31:96–101.

MAGUIRE, P. 1976. "The Psychological and Social Sequelae of Mastectomy. In J. G. Howells, ed. *Modern Perspectives in Psychiatric Aspects of Surgery.* New York: Brunner and Mazel, pp. 390–421.

MEYEROWITZ, B. E. 1980. "Psychosocial Correlates of Breast Cancer and Its Treatments." *Psychological Bulletin* 87:108–131.

MORRIS, T., H. S. GREER, AND P. WHITE. 1977. "Psychological and Social Adjustment to Mastectomy: A Two-Year Follow-up Study." *Cancer* 40:2381–2387.

NICHOLS, D. 1982. "Primary Treatment of Breast Cancer." *Clinical Obstetrics and Gynecology* 25:425–431.

NORTHOUSE, L. L. 1981. "Mastectomy Patients and Fear of Cancer Recurrence." *Cancer Nursing* 4:213–220.

PETERS-GOLDEN, H. 1982. "Breast Cancer: Varied Perceptions of Social Support in the Illness Experience." *Social Science and Medicine* 16:483–491.

POLIVY, J. 1977. "Psychological Effects of Mastectomy on a Woman's Feminine Self-Concept." *Journal of Nervous and Mental Disease* 164:77–87.

QUINT, J. C. 1963. "The Impact of Mastectomy." *American Journal of Nursing* 63(11):88–92.

SANGER, C. K. AND M. REZNIKOFF. 1981. "A Comparison of the Psychological Effects of Breast-Saving Procedures with the Modified Radical Mastectomy." *Cancer* 48:2341–2346.

SCHMITT, F. E. 1982. *"The Structuring of a Life Transition Following a Spinal Cord Injury."* Unpublished doctoral dissertation, University of Illinois at the Medical Center, Chicago.

TAYLOR, S. E., R. R. LICHTMAN, J. V. WOOD, A. Z. BLUMING, G. M. DOZIK, AND R. L. LEIBOWITZ. 1985. "Illness-Related and Treatment-Related Factors in Psychological Adjustment to Breast Cancer." *Cancer* 55:2506–2513.

WESTLAKE, S. K. 1985. *" Life Transition: Women's Responses to the Experience of Breast Cancer and Mastectomy."* Unpublished master's thesis, University of Wisconsin-Milwaukee, Milwaukee.

WOODS, N. F. AND J. A. EARP. 1978. "Women with Cured Breast Cancer." *Nursing Research* 27:279–285.

WORDEN, J. W. AND A. D. WEISMAN. 1977. "The Fallacy in Postmastectomy Depression." *American Journal of Medical Sciences* 273:169–175.

14

The Social Context of Breast Cancer Within the Family

Alice L. Cullinan, PhD

Little attention has been paid to the social context of the female mastectomy patient in professional literature (Spiegel, Bloom, and Gottheil 1983). As a result, the literature on families of patients with breast cancer is largely descriptive, emphasizing a variety of therapeutic interventions. The breast cancer patient has most often been studied in isolation, separate from family and social interaction. This is despite the fact that breast cancer is a life-threatening illness that can impel the woman to rely on family resources and that disrupts the marital dyad and family system. In this essay, I will discuss the relationship between various dimensions of the family environment and patient adjustment to breast cancer.

For ten years, I have worked as a therapist assisting cancer patients to cope with life and death. The work has been done individually, within the marital dyad, the family system or the therapeutic group. In that time, I have had exquisite teachers: the patients and families themselves. They have taught me that deep within the human person and within the family are rich coping resources which, if tapped, can enable the person and family to become stronger and find meaning in the midst of meaninglessness.

According to Taylor, Lichtman and Wood (1984), breast cancer is a major cause of death among American women, striking approximately one out of every eleven women. However, because the survival rate is continually improving, currently 87 percent of the victims of localized breast cancer survive past five years. Because so many women are living substantial numbers of years with the aftermath of illness and treatment, understanding the psychosocial factors that influence the quality of that life is an important issue. Among the factors I will explore here will be: (1) the need for social support systems; (2)

the marital dyad, including issues of communication and sexuality; (3) the family system, including female and male children; (4) therapeutic interventions; and (5) areas for future research.

SOCIAL SUPPORT NEEDS

"The understanding of the problems of any patient with cancer cannot be divorced from an understanding of her social network and environment" (Goldberg and Tull 1983, p. 1). Vachon and Lyall (1976) had previously written that many of the most difficult problems of cancer patients involved reaction to their disease by families and others in their social milieu. Social isolation and the withdrawal of social support can be severely stressful for these patients at a time when they are most in need of the loving care of those closest to them. Fears of "contagion" are not uncommon, even in significant others.

Ostchega and Jacob (1984) demonstrated that the mastectomy patient's social support system is crucial in the adjustment to the illness. They discussed a common problem that occurs with mastectomy patients, who often have a passive-defending coping style that attracts less social support and can give the illusion that there are no unmet emotional needs. Nerenz (1979) found that patients often reported changes in their relationships with family and friends after the surgery. They feel they are avoided or overprotected, unable to communicate their thoughts and feelings about cancer-related issues. When I first started working with cancer patients, I was temporarily led astray because so many of them wanted to talk about how *I* was and seemed to have no need to talk about themselves. I soon learned that beneath this facade there was hurt, panic, and anxiety—all hidden from significant others, friends, medical personnel, and even the patient herself.

Researchers have speculated that one probable cause of problems with family support is actual or perceived rejection by the spouse or other family members, especially since the cancer produces a visible deformity.

Why do women with mastectomies not work harder to fight the feelings of rejection? Most times, the reason is depression (Meyerowitz 1980), which the woman attempts to rationalize away by saying, "There is nothing to discuss" or " They have their own problems, I don't want to burden them" (Frank-Stromberg and Wright, 1984 p. 124). Nevertheless, the nature and availability of support from family, friends, and health personnel are especially important in cancer because of the stigma and misunderstanding surrounding the illness.

When good social support is available, as Morris, Greer, and White (1977) found in 24 percent of the women they surveyed, patients will survive longer than expected (Parkes 1975). Weisman and Worden (1975), in commenting on this finding, wrote that the implications are clear: if the patient and family can be helped to come to terms with the illness and to stay close to each other, life can be prolonged. Jamison, Wellisch, and Posnau (1978) likewise found that better adjustment in mastectomy patients after surgery is correlated with increased emotional support. Conversely, Bloom (1982) reported that patients' perceptions of lack of social support was correlated with levels of emotional distress over the disease and adjuvant therapy. In their study of 238 breast cancer patients, Ward et al (1985) found that patients who felt they received less support than they wanted reported higher distress than did those who did not feel they received less support than they wanted. In addition, lack of social support was "clearly related" (p. 15) in the study to the degree of difficulty patients had with chemotherapy. Murawski, Penman, and Schmitt (1978) wrote that social support is identified as a protective factor buffering the effects of stressor factors in coping with the disease.

How does social support work in helping the woman? Smith et al (1985) addressed this issue. They believed that a positive sense of social support may favor behavioral adjustment to a functional loss and to the threat of death.

Dunkel-Schetter (1984) cautioned that some types of support offered were not well received by the women they studied. Advice and information from family and friends were seen as unhelpful and even bothersome. Understanding which sources are best able to provide the different types of support in the specific situation of mastectomy aftermath is "of paramount importance" (p. 89). Funch and Marshall (1984) wrote that the relationship between social support, stress, and outcome was modified by a self-reliance factor in the mastectomy patients they studied. Generally, they said, social support seemed more positively related to adjustment among other-reliant individuals than self-reliant ones. Therefore, a woman who feels in personal control may neither need nor want as much social support.

Smith et al (1985) found that the primary social support for 87 percent of the women in their study was the husband, followed by friends and children. What of the support persons themselves? What effect does their role have on their ability to function? Klein (1973) posed this question as she asked how many families weather the crisis of cancer successfully. How many husbands, guilty at their inability to help the patient, resign themselves to a vitiated and often destructive marriage? How many children develop school problems in response to an unexplained and mysterious depression in their mothers? I will address these issues from the viewpoints of both the patient and the significant others.

MARITAL INTERACTION

I found no data to suggest that never-married or currently unmarried women suffered more psychosocial distress as a result of mastectomy than do currently married women. In fact, Metzger and Rogers (1983) reported that being married actually intensified the emotional consequences of mastectomy, especially for older (over age 50) women, rather than protecting against them. A number of studies have attempted to assess the impact of breast cancer diagnosis and subsequent surgery on the marital dyad. I found conflicting results. Lee and Maguire (1975) described an increasing incidence of marital discord and sexual problems, and a diminution in leisure and social activity for married couples. Smith et al (1985) reported that husbands seemed to be available for emotional closeness and to be able to provide an adequate amount of support. They also found that for married women, the most important type of support was the husband's listening to, or talking with, the patient about the disease. The findings also included information that the more education husband and wife had about the disease, especially before the surgery, the better able they were to adapt. The study by Smith et al was limited because it was done shortly after diagnosis and there was no follow-up.

The research of Cohen and Wellish (1978) revealed that the husband often feels displaced by his wife's cancer. "Cancer is like the main member of this family now, an unwelcome member that has moved me out and taken over" (p. 5). Wellisch, Mosher, and Van Scay (1978) wrote that husbands are very concerned and troubled by mastectomy in their spouses, but that a significant subgroup of them deny any problem and are unable to cope with their wives' conflicts and problems. My clinical experience is that such husbands will tend to bury themselves in their work. Gotay's (1984) work found that fear of reoccurrence of cancer is the primary fear of both wives and husbands. Men are much more worried about their wives dying than the wives themselves are.

Effects on Sexual Behavior

In his symbolic interactionist interpretation of sexual arousal, Victor (1978) analyzed the relationship between bodily functioning and social learning in erotic behavior. Bodily factors provide the potential for sexual arousal, he said, but it is ultimately learned and interpersonal factors that activate that possibility. Victor applied the social learning model in which conditioning, modeling, and cognitive learning are the fundamentals to sexual behavior and provide the social/psychological mechanisms of erotic response.

The sociologist wrote that in relation to the perception of erotic meanings, the "great American breast fetish" (p. 160) must be considered. Kinsey found, in his research on male sexuality, that there is reason to believe more males in our culture are psychically aroused by contemplation of the female breast than by the sight of the female genitalia. Many American men believe that all women are sexually aroused by breast caressing, and that large-breasted women are more sexually responsive than are small-breasted women. Neither is true. Victor explained how he thought that at an early age, when sexual intercourse would evoke feelings of guilt and embarrassment, American teenagers commonly practiced breast fondling as a substitute for genital contact. Breast fondling during petting reinforces the erotic significance of women's breasts. Yet, in many societies, women are publicly bare-chested without having to be concerned about evoking sexual arousal in men. In many societies, the female breast is a symbol of motherhood and maternal nurturance (unreplaced by bottle feeding). However, in American society, women who have breast-fed their babies in public have been arrested for public sexual indecency. The percentage of American mothers who breast-feed their babies is among the lowest in the world. It is clear that women's breasts are a sexual rather than a maternal symbol among Americans. In American culture, there has arisen a veritable breast cult composed of training bras, padded bras, bustline exercises, and silicone treatments. Many young women suffer anxiety about their breast size and worry about their attractiveness to men.

Victor speculates that the female breast is so important as an erotic symbol in American culture because it is an obvious physical symbol of feminine identity. It has become a prestige symbol as well. Many Americans worry about the degree of their masculinity or feminity. In sharp contrast to increasing similarities between the sexes in behavior and clothing styles, women's breasts visually signal women's distinctiveness from men. Well-developed breasts symbolically reassure women of their feminine attractiveness. In a complementary way, men learn to be erotically attracted to that symbol of female sexuality, often confusing quantity with quality.

Schwain (1976) wrote that to understand how mastectomy affects a women and her partner, it is important to ascertain:

(1) How critical is her perception of her breasts to her self-image and sexual identity?
(2) How significant is the breast in terms of her sexual arousal and gratification?
(3) If she is a mother, did she breast feed?
(4) What impact does a mastectomy have on herself, not only as a sexual person but also as the nurturing woman?

Sexual Functioning

Meyerowitz (1980) wrote that there is little substantive data about the decrease in orgasmic response or frequency of sexual contact following mastectomy. Recent studies do suggest evidence of distress associated with sexual issues subsequent to radical breast surgery and the fact that women's sexual self-image, attitudes, and actual behaviors change following this loss.

Zilbergeld (1979) suggested several reasons why health care providers fail to give serious consideration to the sexual issues faced by chronically ill persons: (1) sex is viewed as an area not vital to revovery and the maintenance of good health; (2) health care providers are not comfortable or not competent confronting sexual issues; and (3) physicians frequently assume that the causes of sexual dysfunction are disease-based, with psychological reactions of the patient and family rarely considered as contributing to sexual difficulties.

The work of Glaser and Strauss (1967) is valuable in understanding the value of renormalizing the sense of one's physical self as a step in the process of adaptation to disease. Anderson and Wolf (1986) cite their work in arguing that diagnosis can begin an eroding of sexual identity and loss of self-esteem if sexual adaptations are not made. These adaptations, the specifics of which I found nothing in the literature, can, in my clinical experience, best be made through communication (1) with another woman who has undergone the trauma; (2) with her husband, as questions of sexuality and relationship are discussed; (3) in support groups; and (4) with her physician.

The literature suggests that breast loss is the central emotional crisis of breast cancer (Silberfarb, Maurere, and Crouthamel 1980). A study by Taylor et al of 209 breast cancer patients (1985) revealed a significantly higher affectional and sexual relationship with husbands for women who had chosen lumpectomy over mastectomy (with no adverse reactions to their health). The more radical the surgery, the more negatively affected were the woman and the marital relationship. In addition, the study showed that reconstructed women were better adjusted than nonreconstructed women. These findings were validated by those of Steinberg, Juliano, and Wise (1985), who found that two years after surgery, lumpectomy patients reported feeling as attractive and feminine as before surgery, whereas mastectomy patients did not. The lumpectomy patients also reported that their husband's sexual behavior had intensified after the surgery, whereas the mastectomy patients perceived a decline in their spouses' sexual interest. In writing about the male perspective, Wellisch, Jamison and Posnau (1980) said that 10 percent of spouses of mastectomy patients, but no spouses of lumpectomy patients, were experiencing severe sexual difficulty 14 months after surgery. In addition, the authors reported significantly better postsurgical sexual adjustment for both types of surgery when there was a high quality of presurgical marital relationship. Meyerowitz (1980) wrote that simple decrease in coital activity was the single most distressing event for women with breast cancer. This, coupled with the report of cancer patients' need for increased physical closeness, intensifies the need for physicians to overcome their own shyness and openly question patients about marital and sexual functioning. The physician need not be an expert, as supportive listening is often all that is needed.

Often, there is a need after breast surgery for a physiological assessment of female sexual arousal function. Barlow (1986), in writing of the role of anxiety, depression, and cognitive interference on sexual dysfunction after mastectomy, showed how fear of inadequacy can lead to cognitive processes that significantly influence sexual arousal. He suggested treatment focused on cognitive change and allocation of attention. However, he cautioned that performance-based exercises may still be the most effective way to restore functioning.

LoPiccolo and LoPiccolo (1978) recommended the use of the masturbation program they developed for the treatment of sexual dysfunction arising after mastectomy. It is based on a sexual-skills learning model. They said that the factor that appears to determine treatment success is marital happiness prior to the onset of the disease. Secondary inorgasmic women respond better when traditional marital therapy is combined with sex therapy.

Importance of Communication

A useful way in which to understand communication changes that can occur in a marriage as a result of breast cancer is through a theory known as symbolic interactionism. Stryker (1967a) wrote that as a social psychological theory, symbolic interactionism addresses a number of related questions, most of which can be seen in the context of two major problems: (1) socialization: how the human organism acquires the ways of behaving or the values, norms, and attitudes of the social units of which one is a part; and (2) personality or the organization of persistent behavior problems. Stryker wrote that the task of social psychology is to account for such organization insofar as it depends on social organizations. Even though he cautioned that ''symbolic interactionism addresses itself largely to the normal person in the sense of the person without gross physical, physiological, or psychological defect'' (p. 372), I find the theory valuable in exploring communication within systems affected by this very gross invasion. In symbolic interactionism, the basic unit of observation is the interaction; from that interaction, both society and the individual derive. According to this theory, the self is defined in terms of socially recognized categories and their corresponding roles. Since these roles necessarily imply relationship, the self necessarily implies relations. One's self is, then, the way one describes to oneself relationships to others in a social process.

Role taking is an important concept in this theory and refers to anticipating the responses of others implicated with one in some social act. This role taking is obviously related to such concepts as empathy, insight, and social sensitivity. Stryker (1967b) wrote that vulnerability increases the likelihood of blocks to communication. However, he said that ignorance can be viewed as an active and often positive element in operating structures and role relationships. Studies show that this is very much so for management of the fears in coping with cancer. Women fare best in terms of adjustment, remission, and longevity rates who can adequately use denial of the possibility of death in a way that does not interfere with medical treatment but enables them to get on with the business of living. However, as will be seen shortly, this can present difficulties for marital and family functioning. According to Stryker, role-taking as understood in his theory of symbolic interactionism may involve the accurate anticipation and functioning of responses of some particular significant other. Therefore, it would seem that one's role as wife, mother, and even woman will be a function of the extent to which one is defined by significant others as such. Crisis will always threaten identifications, for they depend on stable activities of others with reference to oneself, and crises are likely to be important in the process by which identities change. These changes take place according to the type of awareness contexts present. Hewitt (1976) wrote that description and analysis of awareness contexts are essential to a full understanding of how people interact. In general, when awareness contexts are not open, considerable energies are devoted either to opening them up or keeping them closed. Not only is it the relationship, but also the situation that is being defined by the particular awareness context. Glaser and Strauss (1967) discuss four types of awareness contexts. For my purposes here, I will mention only two—pretense awareness and closed awareness—because they are often present in marriages and families where cancer is present.

Pretense awareness context occurs when both interactants are fully aware but pretend not to be. An example of this is a couple I am working with. Joan and Tom are in their middle thirties and Joan, who has been diagnosed as having mammary carcinoma, stage III, has had a double mastectomy. Immediately after the surgery, the physician sat down separately with each and told them there was a 65 percent possibility of recurrence. In separate sessions with each, I learned that both thought almost constantly of a recurrence and eventual death: however, they had never discussed it. Only after both were helped to communicate their fears and anxieties could they live with a fully aware context—living each day to the fullest and working together towards Joan's health.

In closed awareness, when one interactant does not know either the other's identity or view of the identity, there is the possibility of erosion of the marriage itself. The husband is not aware, for example, of his wife's feelings of diminished feminity and sexual inadequacy or concerns about her changed role in the home. Therefore, there cannot be open communication. Nuehring and Barr (1980) referred to this when they wrote that a husband's innocent actions, such as the use of protectiveness and caution in making sexual advances, may be misread as rejection by a wife who sees her mastectomy as a severe insult to her feminity and sexual desireability (p. 53).

Some years ago, Josephine was referred to me by the American Cancer Society because she was seriously depressed. She had had a double mastectomy and even though she had survived cancer beyond five years, she felt "like a second class citizen" in the home because of the sick/wellness role (Meyerowitz 1980) that she assumed and also had imposed on her in the home. In addition, she was struggling with feelings of disfigurement, which Quint (1963) found can persist for years and are related to depression. There had been no sexual intimacy in the home between her husband and herself since the surgeries. Whenever she broached the subject with him, he would say, "Stop bitching, you're alive, aren't you?" When I saw Bill, three months into the therapy, he seemed an example of what Sattler (1976) named the inexpressive male who does not indicate affection, tenderness, or emotion and does not use behavior that is supportive of the affective expectations of one's wife. Sattler claimed that the function of this behavior is to preserve power, and I believe that this was the case with Bill. Only after I brought the five children into therapy and enabled them to verbalize their fears and anxieties was enough pressure brought to bear on Bill that he could begin to speak of his feelings of anxiety, loneliness, and panic about what would happen to him and the children if Josephine died. Incidentally, this was the first time I met daughters who were afraid of "catching" their mother's breast cancer (this will be discussed below).

Atwater (1982) stressed the importance of awareness within the marital dyad, but nowhere in the literature did I find its application to homes in which there was serious illness. Glaser and Strauss (1967) do discuss it in terms of families in which there is a dying member.

THE FAMILY SYSTEM

When cancer hits, said Olsen (1970), the family and not just the patient has the illness. "Cancer invades a family in much the same way that it invades a human body "(Parkes 1975, p. 1271). Olsen (1970) found that cancer frequently creates a crisis in the family; Wellisch, Moscher, and Van Scay (1978) demonstrated that families function in a perpetual psychological limbo in relation to the disease. They quote a spouse saying "cancer is like another member of our family, an unwelcome member" (p. 228) and conclude that families have to adjust to a new psychological family homeostasis to accommodate the new member. The family's interactions, plans, goals, and finances often become unbalanced (Cohen and Wellisch 1978) and can remain so indefinitely. Today, because of modern medical practice, cancer has changed from an acute to a chronic catastrophe. Parkes' (1975) idea of psychosocial transition was used by Mages and Mendolsohn (1979) in conceptualizing the long-term and evolving effects of cancer. A common element is that the passage through a period of crisis leads to an altered state in which values, time perspective, social roles, and self-image may be permanently changed. The person and family enter what can meaningfully be called a new stage of life as a consequence of the crisis. "There is, we believe, good reason to conclude that the effects of cancer typically persist indefinitely in the family" (Mages and Mendolsohn 1979, p. 259).

In 1980, Nuehring and Barr wrote that in the area of research, a great need existed for the investigation of the sociopsychological impact of breast cancer on patients. They stated that there were many gaps in current knowledge of the impact of a patient's illness on family and friends. The role which significant others play in a patient's recovery, coping, and adjustment, and the extent to which they are at high risk of experiencing psychological distress, are only beginning to be understood. Schnaper (1978) wrote that families play an integral part as the cancer patient moves through different phases of the disease. He showed how family reactions directly and indirectly affect the patient and the helpers.

Ringer (1979) demonstrated how coping with breast cancer brought her family closer: ". . . just quietly holding each other close, in spite of IV's, nose tubes and all the rest meant so much. We were close then, but my illness made us even closer" (p. 65).

Parkes (1975) believed that patients and family members are faced with the need to undergo a process of realization: the need to abandon one view of the world—a view which has been built up and elaborated over many years of their lives—and to substitute another, more appropriate view. "These psychosocial transitions take time and energy" (p. 1272).

Since I view all families as social systems, I see any change in one part of the system causing changes in all other components of that system. Several authors have given evidence that supports my view: Lichtman et al (1984) reported that over twenty cancer researchers and clinicians (whom they name) have observed that members of a patient's family can be severely affected when a patient is diagnosed and treated for cancer. The reactions of the family members are important, both in their own right and because family members may not be able to provide support for the patient unless they are able to work through their difficulties in coping with the situation.

Wellisch, Moscher and Van Scay (1978) reported that families who experience the greatest difficulties in coping with cancer and who are most prone to develop serious psychosomatic or psychological symptomatology are those in which one of the members has had significant psychological difficulties previously. The inability to adjust emotionally to cancer is not a unitary phenomenon, but the latest example of long-term difficulties in the family system, especially in adjusting to life changes. However, given the best of family systems, cancer in a family member dramatically alters the social patterns of that system.

Edstrom and Miller (1981) illustrated how Burr's family stress theory provides a model for examining the family system under stress and for guiding interventions. In the basic model, the crisis is determined by the interaction of the stress event, the family's perception of the event and the family's resources. In intervention, each element is examined separately and efforts are made to achieve a more efficient homeostasis.

Most persons and families react to the diagnosis of cancer with initial feelings of shock and depersonalization. When the word *cancer* is heard, the most frequent psychological association is that of death (McCollum 1978). After the initial reaction of shock, a period of denial and minimalization usually ensues. Denial seems to be an almost universal response, but it can occur along a continuum from momentary regrouping of ego defenses to a serious problem of treatment avoidance.

Philbin (1981) discussed how lack of authentic interactions in a cancer-present family can render the ill person interpersonally dead and may lead to a self-perception by the patient of one who is fading from genuine human experience. This can be compounded by her trying to deal with what Simonton (1984) called the ''secret wish''—family members wishing the ordeal was over.

In addition, both patient and family face numerous difficult decisions. Choices must be made between types of surgery, kinds of adjuvant therapy, and which doctor's advice to heed. The difficulty of decision-making will be compounded by shifts in attention of different family members from immediate to remote threats and back again, which lead to differences in the way the disease and its implications for the family are represented by different members. Kaplan (1977) showed how each participant in the drama will represent the problem from his or her own perspective and develop coping resources relevant to that perception. If the cancer crisis is focused and well-defined, and as long as the medical staff facilitates this clarity with adequate communication, the representations formed by patient and family should show substantial overlap, thus facilitating the development of coping plans and actions that integrate individual roles into a relatively effective and harmonious whole. The occurrence of chronic illness in an adult member of a family can lead to an increase in its cohesiveness and in a sense of well-being of its members (Boss 1986).

Simonton (1984) taught that the open expression of feelings within a family is so crucial to the overall health of its members that a great deal of attention must be placed on this. The reason for her emphasis is that ''communicating feelings within the family is paramount in creating a healing atmosphere and helping the patient gain the psychological strength to work toward recovery'' (p. 139). Simonton teaches that communication is a matter of learned behavior and gives many ways this learning can be facilitated. I recommend a reading of her book to anyone interested in how families can contribute to the healing of cancer in one of their members.

The Children

Kerr (1981) used a family system theory to illustrate how, in a dysfunctional family, an exaggerated use of anxiety-binding mechanisms can result in emotional distancing, with the spouses and children all being cut off from each other. When this occurs, anxieties and lack of differentiation are focused on one or more of the children, and this interferes with their functioning. At times of high family anxiety, these overinvolved children are the most vulnerable to emotional or social dysfunctions.

Although there have been studies on the impact of cancer on a patient's spouse, the reactions of a cancer patient's children have received less attention. Investigators who have explored this area highlight potential problems. Buckley (1977) interviewed 40 families in which one of the parents had advanced cancer and found that during the parent's illness, behavioral disorders in the children increased 33 percent. Typical behaviors of these troubled children were problems in school, withdrawal from peers, increased aggression, night terrors, appetite disturbances, and antisocial problems.

Wellisch (1979) suggested that in response to a mother's cancer, adolescents may demonstrate such acting-out behavior as running away from home, withdrawal from family and friends, a marked drop in school performance, stealing, drug abuse, and promiscuity. In a later study, Wellisch (1981) specifically addressed the home of a breast cancer patient. Drawing from his clinical observations, he noted that breast cancer can produce both overt changes for children (such as the child needing to take on extra household responsibilities) and covert changes (such as shifts in roles for the adolescent in relation to both the sick mother and the well father). Providing nurturant support for the ill parent may be beyond the child's developmental repertoire. Thus, new role requirements can lead to more intense emotional involvement between an adolescent and an ill parent, and such demands may conflict with the adolescent's developmental need for gradual emotional withdrawal from the family. Adolescents who find themselves in such a conflictual bind may respond by acting out.

Wellisch (1981) indicated that the relationship between a mother who has had a mastectomy and her adolescent daughter may be especially vulnerable to discord. He surmised that the mother's distress may stem from her envy of her daughter's intact body, which may promote feelings of rivalry between the two and may lead to sexual acting-out by the daughter. Lichtman et al (1984) reported that the fear of inheriting breast cancer and the mother's demand on the daughter for support were judged to be major contributing factors to the difficulties with adolescent and postadolescent daughters.

INTERVENTIONS

There is a substantial amount of literature on interventions for breast cancer patients, their spouses, families and children. Here I will only mention some of the outstanding ones in which I have been involved. Meyerowitz (1980) wrote of the number of authors who have recommended combining the sources of support available by providing multidisciplinary groups for cancer patients and their families. Cohen and Wellisch (1978) have written of the efficacy of the use of family therapy, using the systems approach. Bloom and Spiegel (1984) lauded the use of any social-support interventions, "whether individual counseling or peer support groups," that improved psychological well being and decreased feelings of powerlessness. Klein (1973) discussed some ways in which the breast patient and her family can be helped to perform the psychological tasks essential to healthy coping. For both patient and family, they include: (1) help in the expression of feelings; (2) help in sorting out the real from the unreal; (3) refusal to give false reassurances; (4) help in anticipating the future; (5) helping the family to understand the patient's feelings and to express theirs; and (6) helping the patient to consider how and what to tell those significant persons in her life.

AREAS FOR FUTURE RESEARCH

Well-designed longitudinal studies of breast cancer patients and their families are needed. These studies could follow the reactions and adjustment of subjects over time, from diagnosis to treatment to follow-up after treatment. Cross-ethnic surveys that explore people's perceptions of breast cancer and its surgical and chemotherapeutic treatment are also in order.

An area I am particularly interested in is training of helping professionals to cope more effectively with and provide support for breast cancer patients and their families. If outcome studies can predict what types of enabling activities are most beneficial for patients and their families, then the next task would be to adequately train medical personnel and mental health workers in preventive methodology, crisis intervention, and more long-term counseling techniques.

REFERENCES

ANDERSON, B. AND F. WOLF. 1986. "Chronic Physical Illness and Sexual Behavior: Psychological Issues." *Journal of Consulting and Clinical Psychology* 54: 168–175.

ATWATER, L. 1982. *The Extramarital Connection; Sex, Intimacy and Identity.* New York: Irvington Press.

BARLOW, D. 1986. "Causes of Sexual Dysfunction: The Role of Anxiety and Cognitive Interference." *Journal of Consulting and Clinical Psychology* 54: 140-148.

BLOOM, J. 1982. "Social Support, Accomodation to Stress and Adjustment to Cancer." *Social Science and Medicine* 16:1329-1338.

BLOOM, J. AND SPIEGEL, D. 1984. "The Relationship of Two Dimensions of Social Support to the Psychological Well-Being and Social Functioning of Women with Advanced Breast Cancer." *Social Science and Medicine* 19:831-837.

BOSS, P. 1986. "Family Stress Perception and Context." In M. B. Sussman and S. Steinmetz, eds., *Handbook on Marriage and Family.* New York: Plenum Press.

BUCKLEY, I. 1977. *Listen to the Children.* New York: Cancer Care.

COHEN, M. AND D. WELLISCH. 1978. "Living in Limbo: Psychosocial Intervention in Families with a Cancer Patient." *American Journal of Psychotherapy* 32:561-571.

DUNKEL-SCHETTER, C. 1984. "Social Support and Cancer: Findings Based on Patient Interviews and Their Implications." *Journal of Social Issues* 40:77-98.

EDSTROM, S. AND M. MILLER. 1981. "Preparing the Family to Care for the Cancer Patient at Home: A Home Care Course." *Cancer Nursing* 7:49-52.

FRANK-STROMBERG, M. AND P. WRIGHT. 1984. "Ambulatory Cancer Patients' Perception of the Physical and Psychosocial Changes in Their Lives Since the Diagnosis of Cancer." *Cancer Nursing* 7: 117-130.

FUNCH, D. AND J. MARSHALL. 1984. "Self-reliance as a modifier of the Effects of Life Stress and Social Support." *Journal of Psychosomatic Research* 28:9-15.

GLASER, B. AND A. STRAUSS. 1967. "Awareness Contexts and Social Interaction." In J. Manis and B. Meltzer, eds. *Symbolic Interaction: A Reader in Social Psychology.* Boston: Allyn and Bacon.

GOLDBERG, R. AND R. TULL. 1983. *The Psychosocial Dimensions of Cancer Treatment.* New York: Macmillan.

GOTAY, C. 1984. "The Experience of Cancer During Early and Advanced Stages: The Views of Patients and Their Mates." *Social Science and Medicine* 18: 605-613.

HEWITT, J. 1976. *Self and Society: A Symbolic Interactionist Social Psychology.* Boston: Allyn and Bacon.

JAMISON, K. R., D. K. WELLISCH, AND R. POSNAU. 1978. "Psychosocial Aspects of Mastectomy I: The Woman's Perspective." *American Journal of Psychiatry* 135: 432-436.

KAPLAN, D. 1977. "Family Mediation of Stress." In R. H. Moos, ed. *Coping with Physical Illness.* New York: Plenum Press.

KERR, M. 1981. "Cancer and the Family Emotional System." In J. Goldberg, ed. *The Psychotherapeutic Treatment of Cancer Patients.* New York: Macmillan.

KLEIN, R. 1973. "A Crisis to Grow On." *Cancer* 33:1660-1665.

LEE, P. AND R. MAGUIRE. 1975. "Emotional Distress in Patients Attending a Breast Clinic." *British Journal of Surgery* 62: 160-168.

LICHTMAN, R. ET AL. 1984. " Relations with Children after Breast Cancer: The Mother-Daughter Relationship at Risk." *Journal of Psychosocial Oncology* 2:1-19.

LOPICCOLO, J. AND M. LOPICCOLO. 1978. *Handbook of Sex Therapy.* New York: Plenum Press.

MCCOLLUM, P. 1978. "Adjustment to Cancer; A Psychosocial and Rehabilitative Perspective." *Rehabilitation Counseling Bulletin* 218-223.

MAGES, N. AND G. MENDELSOHN. 1979. "The Effects of Cancer on Patients' Lives: A Personological Approach." In G. C. Stone et al., eds. *Health Psychology: A Handbook.* San Francisco: Jossey-Bass, pp. 255-284.

METZGER, L. AND T. ROGERS. 1983. "The Effects of Age and Marital Status on Emotional Distress After a Mastectomy." *Journal of Psychosocial Oncology* 1(3): 17–33.

MEYEROWITZ, B. 1980. "The Psychological Correlates of Breast Cancer and Its Treatment." *Psychological Bulletin* 87: 108–131.

MORRIS, T., S. GREER, AND P. WHITE. 1977. "Psychological and Social Adjustment to Mastectomy." *Cancer* 40: 2381–2387.

MURAWSKI, B., D. PENMAN, AND M. SCHMITT. 1978. "Social Support in Health and Illness." *Cancer Nursing* 4: 365–371.

NERENZ, P. 1979. *Control of Emotional Distress in Cancer Chemotherapy.* Unpublished doctoral dissertation, University of Wisconsin, Madison.

NEUHRING, E. AND W. BARR. 1980. "Mastectomy: Impact on Patients and Families." *Health and Social Work* 5: 53–58.

OLSEN, E. 1970. "The Impact of Serious Illness on the Family System." *Post-Graduate Medicine* 23: 169–174.

OSTCHEGA, J. AND K. JACOB. 1984. "Providing Safe Conduct: Helping Your Patient Cope with Cancer." *Nursing* 4: 43–48.

PARKES, C. 1975. "The Emotional Impact of Cancer on Patients and Families." *Journal of Laryngology and Otology* 89: 1271–1279.

PHILBIN, M. 1981. "The Mysterious Case of Ichabod Crane." In J. Goldberg, ed. *Psychotherapeutic Treatment of Cancer Patients.* New York: Free Press.

RINGER, L. 1979. "A Cancer Patient's Message to Physicians." *Medical Times* 106: 64–67.

QUINT, J. 1963. "The Impact of Mastectomy." *American Journal of Nursing* 63: 88–92.

SATTLER, J. 1976. "The Inexpressive Male: Tragedy or Sexual Politics." *Social Problems* 23: 469–477.

SCHNAPER, N. 1978. "Psychological Roles in the Cancer Drama." *American Journal of the Medical Sciences* 276: 248–261.

SCHWAIN, W. 1976. "Psychosocial Issues in Counseling Mastectomy Patients." *Counseling Psychology* 6: 45–49.

SILBERFARB, P., H. MAURERE, AND C. CROUTHAMEL. 1980. "Psychosocial Aspects of Neoplastic Diseases I." *American Journal of Psychiatry* 137: 450–435.

SIMONTON, S. 1984. *The Healing Family.* New York: Bantam Books.

SMITH, E. ET AL. 1985. "Perceptions of Social Support Among Patients with Recently Diagnosed Breast, Endometrial and Ovarian Cancer." *Journal of Psychosocial Oncology* 3(3): 65–81.

SPIEGEL, D., J. BLOOM, AND E. GOTTHEIL. 1983. "Family Environment as a Predictor of Adjustment to Metastatic Breast Cancer." *Journal of Psychosocial Oncology* 1(1): 33–44.

STEINBERG, D., L. JULIANO, AND L. WISE. 1985. "Psychological Effects of Lumpectomy vs. Mastectomy for Breast Cancer." *American Journal of Psychology* 142: 34–39.

STRYKER, S. 1967a. "Symbolic Interaction as an Approach to Family Research." In J. Manis and B. Meltzer, eds. *Symbolic Interaction: A Reader in Social Psychology.* Boston: Allyn and Bacon, pp. 371–383.

STRYKER, S. 1967b. " Role-taking Accuracy and Adjustment." In J. Manis and B. Meltzer, eds. *Symbolic Interaction: A Reader in Social Psychology.* Boston: Allyn and Bacon, pp. 481–492.

TAYLOR, S., R. LICHTMAN, AND J. WOOD. 1984. "Attributions, Beliefs About Control and Adjustment to Breast Cancer." *Journal of Personality and Social Psychology* 46: 489–502.

TAYLOR, S. ET AL., 1985. "Illness-Related and Treatment-Related Factors to Psychological Adjustment to Breast Cancer." *Cancer* 55: 2506–2513.

VACHON, M. AND W. LYALL. 1976. "Applying Psychiatric Techniques to Patients with Cancer." *Hospital and Community Psychiatry* 27: 582–584.

VICTOR, L. 1978. "A Symbolic Interactionist Interpretation of Sexual Arousal." In N. K. Denzin, ed. *Studies in Symbolic Interaction.* Greenwich, CT: Jai Press.

WARD, S. ET AL. 1985. *Social Support and Distress During Chemotherapy.* Paper delivered at annual meeting of American Psychological Association, San Francisco.

WEISMAN, A. AND J. WORDEN. 1975. *Coping with Vulnerability in Cancer Patients: A Research Report.* Boston: Massachusetts General Hospital.

WELLISCH, D. 1979. "Adolescent Acting Out When a Parent Has Cancer." *International Journal of Family Therapy* 1: 230–241.

WELLISCH, D. 1981. "Family Relationships of the Mastectomy Patient: Interactions with the Spouse and Children." *Israeli Journal of Medical Science* 17: 993–996.

WELLISCH, D., K. JAMISON, AND R. POSNAU. 1980. "Psychological Aspects of Mastectomy II: The Man's Perspective." *American Journal of Psychiatry* 135: 543–546.

WELLISCH, D., M. MOSHER, AND C. VAN SCAY. 1978. "Management of Family Emotion and Stress: Family Group Therapy in a Private Oncology Practice." *Cancer* 47: 345–352.

ZILBERGELD, H. 1979. "Sex and Serious Illness." In C. A. Garfield, ed. *Stress and Survival: The Emotional Realities of Life-Threatening Illness.* St. Louis, MO: C. V. Mosby, pp. 236–242.

15

Existential Group Therapy with Mastectomy Patients

Alice L. Cullinan, PhD

Research reveals that about 30 percent of women with diagnosed breast cancer experience severe psychosocial problems correlated with both the malignancy and the loss of a breast (Stefanek, Derogatis, and Shaw 1986; Farber, Wienerman, and Kuypers 1984; Morris, Greer, and White 1979). After the diagnosis, many women progress through a predictable psychological process, resolving their grief with time and resuming previous life styles with limitation. For others, however, the intervening time can be long and fraught with psychological distress. This chapter addresses the nature of that distress, with its psychosocial variables, and discusses an educational and therapeutic approach for aiding women to cope better with the stress of the disease and its treatment.

PSYCHOLOGICAL PROFILE OF A BREAST CANCER PATIENT

Over 200 articles have addressed the interaction between the psyche and breast cancer before and after diagnosis and treatment. These studies have been appearing for centuries: in 1701 Gendron (reported in Kowal 1955) wrote that while the development of breast cancer was independent of age, marital status, and economic situation, it correlated with sedentary, melancholic, or hysteric dispositions. Since then, authors have implicated many psychological factors in contributing to the development of cancer. These include overwhelming and prolonged stress in one's life (Cooper 1984); a tendency to respond negatively to stress (Kuehn 1986); emotional inhibition (Pettingale, Watson, and Greer 1985); dysfunctional responses to a significant loss and a poor self-image (Simonton, Simonton, and Creighton 1978); a strong tendency to hold

150

resentment or deeply repressed anger (Greer and Morris 1975); a poor ability to develop and maintain long-term meaningful relations (Brown 1966); an inability to express emotions, verbally and repressed sexuality (Wheeler and Caldwell 1955); and use of passivity instead of assertiveness as a coping mechanism (Bacon, Rennecker, and Cutler 1952). Methodological and research design flaws have called into question some of this evidence and for now, the existence of personality variables associated with the development of cancer "continues to warrant further investigation" (Stefanek, Derogatis, and Shaw 1986, p. 538).

EMOTIONAL PROFILE OF POSTMASTECTOMY PATIENTS

More of a consensus exists about the matrix of psychological problems which can erupt in response to breast cancer diagnosis and treatment and the stress of postmastectomy living. Alagaratnam and Kung (1986) found that a positive diagnosis was the most important factor in the psychosocial morbidity of breast cancer patients. The work of Meyerowitz (1980), Harrell (1972), and others, has led to a belief that the emotional trauma resulting from diagnosis and treatment of cancer can be as potentially damaging as the cancer itself. Kushner (1975) found in her worldwide study that a mastectomy can be one of the most emotionally threatening of all surgical procedures, and raises, for many, issues of loss of femininity and sexual attractiveness, necessitating the restructuring of aspects of the patient's premastectomy image.

Sabo, Brown, and Smith (1986) wrote:

> Treatment for breast cancer and aftercare involve considerable psychological and emotional problems . . . mastectomy is apt to result in a major disruption of body image, depression, fears of rejection and death, and deep seated concerns about sexual identity and behavior. (p. 19)

Documented postdiagnostic psychological traumas include "depression, anxiety, anger, and sexual identification and behavior difficulties" (Hill 1986, p. 79), while Peck (1972) believed that absence of emotional impact, an increase in upset over time, or an extremely intense psychotic response to a mastectomy were abnormal responses to diagnosis and treatment. The psychological discomfort experienced immediately after a mastectomy almost always includes depression, anxiety, and anger, often to a severe degree (Derogatis 1977), and it is common for this emotional distress to continue for more than a year following surgery (Maguire 1978).

Gottschalk and Hoigaard-Martin (1986) found that mastectomy patients, when compared with persons with no illness or with other types of cancer, had significantly higher total anxiety, death and mutilation anxiety, ambivalent hostility, and total denial. The mastectomy group also showed more psychopathological emotional responses than the other groups. Changes in psychological responses and patterns of coping often result, especially following surgery. These can include impairment of interpersonal relationships (Dunkel-Schetter and Wortman 1982), suicidal ideation in a quarter of all patients (Meyerowitz 1980), increased use of tranquilizers and alcohol in 40 percent of all patients (Jamison, Wellisch, and Panau 1978) insomnia (Anstice 1970); breast phantoms experienced by half of all mastectomy patients as long as 10 years after surgery (Jarvis 1967). Jamison, Wellisch, and Panau (1978) found that the trauma had a more profound effect upon younger women. Often concerns about the disfigurement persist for several years (Ray 1978), and this extends to difficulty in revealing the incision site to one's sexual partner (Grandstaff 1976), with "an increasing incidence of marital discord, sexual problems, and a diminution in leisure and social activities" (Maguire 1978, p. 79).

Breast cancer can elicit many fears, anxieties and concerns including those of recurrence (Schain 1976), mutilation (Ray 1978) and death (Robbins 1973). Variables affecting the intensity of these fears include participation in treatment decisions (Owens, Ashcroft, Leinster, and Slade 1987), age and marital status (Metzger, Rogers, and Bauman 1983), nature of the marital and sexual relationship (Witkin 1975) and premorbid personality (Meyerowitz 1980). Two environmental factors having an important impact on the psychosocial adjustment of a cancer patient are time (Milton 1973), and access to emotionally supportive relationships (Kaufman and Micha 1987), including the quality of the patient–physician relationship (Ross 1976). Although the support from the physician–patient dyad was found to be of crucial importance to breast cancer patients (Fellner 1975), less than a third of polled surgeons asked their patients about their feelings concerning the illness and less than 20 percent described as a key aspect of their role discussing with patients their feelings about the mastectomy (Ray, Fisher, and Wisniewski 1986).

THE IMPORTANCE OF GROUP TREATMENT FOR CANCER PATIENTS

Group therapy and self-help groups have been found to be a prominent source of support for breast cancer patients (Kaufman and Micha 1987; Spiegel and Glafkides 1983; Spiegel, Bloom, and Yalom 1981; and Kleiman, Mantell, and Alexander 1977). Ferlic, Goldman, and Kennedy (1979) wrote: "Group counseling of cancer patients has become one of the most potentially effective techniques relating to comprehensive cancer care" (p. 760). This team of researchers demonstrated that a newly diagnosed group of cancer patients can be greatly aided by participation in a structured educational and psychological support group. Parsell and Taglireni (1979) reached similar conclusions as their groups of cancer patients worked through themes of helplessness, anguish over the meaning of life and death, and the coping problems of everyday life. Group participants were relieved of the dependency needs that had been fostered by the sick role, resolved suicidal thoughts, learned to cope with pain and side effects of chemotherapy, and developed better communication skills with relatives and friends. Several specific needs of the cancer patient can best be achieved within the group setting, including teaching of relaxation training (Heinrich and Schag 1984), reduction of anxiety (Vachon and Lkyall 1976), and increase in communication skills (Abrams 1966).

INDICATIONS FOR THERAPEUTIC INTERVENTION WITH GROUP THERAPY

Immediately after undergoing a mastectomy, many women are trying to begin discussing its emotional aspects with their partners, and adjuvant therapy may be beginning. Evidence accumulated by Meyerowitz (1980) suggested that women who undergo chemotherapy may have a more difficult and prolonged emotional recovery than those who do not. Ostchega and Jacob (1984) reported that during the first 100 days following mastectomy, the patient is preoccupied with thoughts and questions about "life, interpersonal relationships, and death. The patient may feel angry, be confused and have both misconceptions and realistic fears" (p. 44). Coping mechanisms will include denial and repression. It is during this time that group therapy can be especially effective in strengthening coping mechanisms, providing social support, and addressing existential issues.

EXISTENTIAL GROUP THERAPY FOR METASTATIC BREAST CANCER PATIENTS

The discovery during surgery that a patient's cancer has metastasized will precipitate a crisis based upon the possibility of a limited life span. Usually, additional support and therapy are indicated. Although several types of group approaches have been used with metastatic breast cancer patients, such as supportive (Spiegel and Glafkides 1983), psychoanalytic/supportive (Goldman 1985), and existential (Spiegel, Bloom, and Yalom 1981), it is this last method that seems particularly suited for this population. Existential therapy is focused on concerns rooted in one's existence. Its objective is "the attainment of authenticity of being in all participants" (Hora 1959, p. 88) and, as Yalom (1980) has shown, learning to live and die well:

> I have been struck by how many of them use their crisis and their
> danger (of dying) as an opportunity for change. They report startling
> shifts, inner changes that can be characterized in no other way than
> personal growth (p. 35).

Yalom wrote at length of his use of death as a catalyst for change and growth within groups. Shaffer and Galinsky (1974) expanded on this existential orientation and its conviction that one's unconscious contains within it forces for courage and creativity as well as for violence and cruelty. They believed that it was important to "let the patient be," in the sense of accepting all aspects of his or her being, both healthy and pathological, including the freedom to resist the therapist and the treatment. A key concept of existentialism is distinguishing between authentic and inauthentic existence. Existential group therapy "can be expected to push inauthentic ways of relating into bolder relief than does the one-to-one relationship, since the presence of other people typically engenders an unusual amount of anxiety" (Shaffer and Galinski 1974, p. 104).

Holt (1979) showed how the neurotic anxiety of group participants can be transformed into existential anxiety by the leader and the group helping the patient to confront the life situation and make active choices, regardless of how painful they are. This can lead to chance-taking and individuation in maintaining one's identity, and learning to develop empathetic relationships with significant individuals in one's life, starting with other group members. In this way, one may choose to overcome the tendency toward passivity and nonbeing, making of inauthentic decisions, and becoming an object and a means to an end for others and vice versa. This is a common problem in the lives of cancer patients. Only by enlargement of the patient's awareness of such tendencies and confrontation of the denial of the constantly changing reality which life presents to everyone, can a person maintain himself or herself as an alive, vital human being. Holt further presented this nonmanipulative way of sharing the patient's life world as creating the freedom for both individual group members and the therapist to experience their mutually shared world.

An underpinning of existentialist therapy comes in part from Sartre's (1947) phrase: "la condition humaine," which denotes that each human is cast into the world without his or her consent and must leave it the same way. In the limited and unpredictable span between, one must make the most of one's potential so as to live meaningfully. The response to this human condition is of ultimate importance in determining one's way of life, and it becomes the steering element of one's existence.

Marram (1978) elucidated an aspect of existential group psychotherapy: "The premise that the nature of becoming is in the awareness of the here and now can direct much of the activity that occurs in groups'' (p. 105). She described the existential group experience as providing a space in which participants could identify with and accept the emergent and growing self through experiences of awareness, until this sense of self is revised to the point that oneself (the ''I'') is the (authentic) one thinking, perceiving, feeling, and doing.

The Leader in Existential Group Therapy

Whitaker and Lieberman (1964) viewed the leader of the existential group as the most experienced patient. He or she has grappled with the meaning of life and death, being and nonbeing, being-in-the-world, existential versus neurotic anxiety, and authentic versus inauthentic existence. Having done this, the therapist's primary responsibility is to initiate and maintain interaction and give permission to face and discuss existential issues such as death, pain, loss, suffering, and meaning. After becoming aware of these existential questions, group members can move forward and begin to resolve them in a personal and authentic way. The existential therapist ''is more willing to reveal both his immediate experience in the session and various aspects of his own past'' (Shaffer and Galinsky 1974, p. 105). The therapist also expresses aspects of her own being so that the same can be elicited from the ''other'' patients and so that an authentic atmosphere for each participant is promoted. The selective authenticity of the therapist accentuates the importance of freedom and spontaneity and conveys a respect for the patient's ability to take responsibility for whatever reactions he or she in turn has to the therapist's revelations. Yalom (1980) wrote that the leader must be ''aware of being generally the only person in the group who, on the basis of past experience, has a relatively clear definition in mind of what constitutes a good work meeting'' (p. 226). Thus, the leader is a guide as well as a model. She demonstrates to the members that learned helplessness is an inauthentic mode of being. Lewis (1982) has shown that this is a very important concept for cancer patients to learn. The leader encourages the members to share their impressions and feelings for other members, and encourages honesty and awareness of responsibility. The therapeutic factor of insistence on the patient's learning that she is ultimately alone and responsible for the meaning of her life has been commented on favorably in Bloch, Crouch, and Reibstein's (1981) review of theoretical, empirical, and clinical research on therapeutic factors in group psychotherapy.

The leader must of course be thoroughly trained in psychological principles, group dynamics, and existential therapy. She should, in addition, be educated in ways of coping with the disease and have knowledge of treatment effects. Klagsbrun (1983) believed that an oncotherapist must have a general knowledge of medicine, pharmacology, and pathology, especially in areas relating to cancer, and should be well-informed on advances in chemotherapy—a difficult task these days! Priority should be placed on conveying knowledge about treatment side effects and the need to help patients live with them as best they can. (For example, one patient found that eating saltine crackers immediately before the beginning of chemotherapy was quite effective in relieving nausea.) The oncotherapist needs to communicate to patients currently undergoing chemotherapy what medical professionals most often do not: that side effects frequently include a loss of sexual interest and drive, a lack of concentration, occasional irrational moments and wandering of the mind, a loss of energy, and most importantly depression. "Treating the invisible scars (of chemotherapy) . . . the loss of interest, the decline in motivation for life in general and for specific projects—requires a tremendous amount of tact and knowledge on the oncotherapist's part" (Klagsbrun 1983, p. 57). In additional an oncotherapist must be prepared to tackle the issue of termination of aggressive treatment by the patient in an honest and authentic way and accept that decision unconditionally.

Helping patients cope with the crisis of cancer will place great strains on the therapist's capacity for compassion (Ostchega and Jacob 1984). The therapist, as role model and leader, must maintain an authentic stance regarding her personal needs. Support must be obtained from other than clients, time taken for oneself, and regular opportunities utilized to acquire spiritual, physical, and emotional nurturance. The therapist must be aware of any indications of burnout, the most common being premature emotional or physical disengagement from the patient.

Goals of the Group

The goals of a group for women who have undergone a mastectomy and have metastatic cancer include addressing and helping them to cope with both existential and practical concerns. Specific apprehensions include: fears of spread of the cancer (Weisman and Worden 1986); fear of and anxiety about death (Ostchega and Jacob 1984); feelings of helplessness (Parsell and Taglireni 1974); inability to verbalize feelings (Worris et al. 1981); lack of felt emotional support (Goldberg and Tull 1983); depression, insomnia, and low motivation (Klagsbrun 1983); issues surrounding sexuality (Maguire 1976); the relationship with the physician (Frank-Stromberg and Wright 1984); education about cancer, treatment, and side effects (Majes and Mendelsohn 1979); and marital problems accelerating after surgery (Metzger, Rogers, and Bauman 1983).

A no less important goal is that of providing social support as a source of coping. Bloom (1982) has written of the importance of this assistance for mastectomy patients in helping them to feel accepted regardless of their condition, by serving as a protection against the potential devastating traumas of the disease and providing interpersonal emotional nurturance and response.

An Example of an Existentially-Oriented Post-mastectomy Group

I share now a model I use in existential group work with women with metastic breast cancer. Ideally, patients selected are within 100 days of having had the mastectomy, are free of psychotic disorders, are desirous of psychotherapeutic intervention, and have permission for participation from their oncologist. Prospective group members are seen individually three times prior to involvement in the group. Yalom (1975) suggested that this brief individual work results in more effective and long-lasting therapeutic change. Mullen and Rosenbaum (1962) demonstrated that during this time the therapist has five functions, which overlap to some degree: (1) history taking, (2) beginning of establishment of the therapeutic relationship, (3) acquainting the patient with the idea of the group, (4) surfacing of major resistances to the idea of group, and (5) orientation toward full participation in an existentially oriented group. After the three preparatory individual sessions, no further individual sessions are usually held with the client, because this would tend to isolate him from potentially therapeutic group experiences and vitiate the critical therapeutic experience for the patient. The groups are closed, meaning that no new members are admitted once membership is established. The parameters include total confidentiality, consistency of meeting time and place (twice weekly in my office), and a set time span for the group. I have found that three months usually allows sufficient time for important issues to be faced and resolved.

Coping with the deterioration and the eventual death of a member is a crisis event for the group, to which group members usually respond by becoming more supportive of one another. The shared experience of "I'm not in this alone" is immensely valuable for participants, who are often astonished to discover that others have fears and concerns similar to theirs. As participants allow deep and often primitive fears, previously unacceptable, to emerge, those fears can be seen more realistically. For example, when an attractive 35-year-old woman verbalized a fear of being abandoned by her husband because of her disfigurement and perceived sexual unattractiveness, other group members were able to admit they had similar fears and encouraged one another to discuss the concern with their spouses. During a subsequent meeting, most shared that the discussions with their husbands had been emotional but positive, and had resulted in feeling greater support and understanding from them. When one member's husband did admit that he was thinking of finding another sexual partner, the group was encouraging to her and recommended marital counseling (in which the couple did become involved). Because so many cancer patients experience difficulty in being assertive, training for assertiveness is also another regular component of the process.

Fear of pain if the cancer spreads is a common topic in the early stages of the group. After allowing participants to express their concerns, I educate them on medications now available that can usually ameliorate pain. In addition, in the early weeks of the group, I teach a relaxation exercise which can help relieve nausea and other iatrogenic side effects of treatment.

Usually between the fifth and eighth week of the sessions, a desire emerges from within the group to learn how "to make the most of the rest of my life." A questioning of the meaning and purpose of one's life occurs, and a focusing on new values and directions often emerges. Issues such as the quality of one's married and family life, other relationships, belief system, and unfulfilled dreams are addressed. One woman had dreamed of going on an ocean cruise, but had always felt constrained by the financial needs of her family. Encouraged by the group, she shared her dream with her husband. They were able to borrow some money and, after the group ended, went on the cruise.

About the tenth week, termination issues begin appearing, often accompanied by a certain anxiety. Participants are encouraged to share these concerns, which often trigger earlier unresolved grief issues. Learning to grieve is an important task for some of the women, and one they have previously denied or repressed. Often anger, a renewed sense of helplessness ("I thought I was over that"), and very real psychic pain emerge. With encouragment and support by the leader and other members, this task can be accomplished rather quickly in most cases. If it cannot, the women are encouraged to seek further therapy. During the twelfth or last session, I ask each participant to share one gift they would want to leave with the others. Some responses have been: "vitality of living," "hope for the future—however long it is to be," "love," "a new belief in myself," "the ability to get mad and know it's OK," "not being afraid to die now," and "a greater sense of closeness to God."

Conclusion

This chapter has surveyed research results of studies on the psychological responses and needs of women with breast cancer and, more specifically, of those with metastasis. It has discussed a particular mode of adjunctive treatment to address those needs and described phenomenologically a group process in which I participate as a leader. Although perhaps not suitable for everyone, this modality nevertheless has the potential for aiding many in the rehabilitation from what can be a traumatic and life-threatening event in a woman's life.

REFERENCES

ABRAMS, T. 1966. "The Patient with Cancer: The Changing Pattern of Communication." *New York Journal of Nursing* 274:317–322.

ALAGARATNAM, T. T. AND N. Y. KUNG. 1986. "Psychosocial Effects of Mastectomy: Is it Due to Mastectomy or to the Diagnosis of Malignancy?" *British Journal of Psychiatry* 149:296–299.

ANSTICE, E. 1970. "Coping After a Mastectomy." *Nursing Times* 66:882–883.

BACON, E., R. RENNECKER, AND M. CUTLER. 1952. "A Psychosomatic Survey of Cancer of the Breast." *Psychosomatic Medicine* 14:453–460.

BLOCH, S., E. CROUCH, AND J. REIBSTEIN. 1981. "Therapeutic Factors in Group Psychotherapy." *Archives of General Psychiatry* 38:519–528.

BLOOM, J. R. 1982. "Social Support, Accommodation to Stress, and Adjustment to Breast Cancer." *Journal of Social Science and Medicine* 16:1329–1338.

BROWN, F. 1966. "The Relationship Between Cancer and Personality." *Annals of the New York Academy of Sciences* 163:865–873.

COOPER, C. L. 1984. "Sociopsychological Precursors to Cancer." In C. L. Cooper, ed. *Psychosocial Stress and Cancer*. New York: John Wiley and Sons, pp. 21–36.

DEROGATIS, L. R. 1977. "Cancer Patients and Their Physicians in the Perception of Psychological Symptoms." *Psychosomatics* 17:197–201.

DUNKEL-SCHETTER, C. AND C. B. WORTMAN. 1982. "The Interpersonal Dynamics of Cancer: Problems in Social Relationships and Their Impact on the Patient." In H. S. Friedman and M. R. DiMatteo, eds. *Interpersonal Issues in Health Care*. New York: Academic Press, pp. 69–100.

FARBER, D. M., B. H. WIENERMAN AND J. A KUYPERS. 1984. "Psychosocial Distress in Oncology Outpatients." *Journal of Psychosocial Oncology* 2:109–118.

FELLNER, C. 1975. "Family Disruption After Cancer Cure." *American Family Physician* 8:169–172.

FERLIC, M., A. GOLDMAN, AND B. KENNEDY. 1979. "Group Counseling in the Adult Patient with Advanced Cancer." *Cancer* 43:760–766.

FRANK-STROMBERG, M. AND P. WRIGHT. 1984. "Ambulatory Cancer Patients: Perception of the Physical and Psychosocial Changes in Their Lives Since the Diagnosis of Cancer." *Cancer Nursing* 7:117–130.

GOLDBERG, R. AND R. TULL. 1983. *Psychosocial Dimensions of Cancer Treatment*. New York: Macmillan.

GOLDMAN, R. A. 1985. "Psychoanalytic and Supportive Approaches in the Postmastectomy Group." *Dynamic Psychotherapy* 3(2):145–155.

GOTTSCHALK, L. A. AND J. HOIGAARD-MARTIN. 1986. "The Emotional Impact of Mastectomy." *Psychiatry Research* 17(2):153–167.

GRANDSTAFF, N. 1976. "The Impact of Breast Cancer on the Family." *Frontiers of Radiation and Oncology* 11:145–156.

GREER, S. H. AND J. MORRIS. 1975. "Psychological Attributes of Women Who Develop Breast Cancer: A Controlled Study." *Journal of Psychosomatic Research* 19:147–153.

HARRELL, H. 1972. "To Lose a Breast." *American Journal of Nursing* 197:676–677.

HEINRICH, R. AND C. SCHAG. 1984. "A Behavioral Medicine Approach to Coping with Cancer." *Cancer Nursing* 7:243–247.

HILL, H. L. 1986. "Radiation or Mastectomy: A Choice for Living." *Journal of Psychosocial Oncology* 4(1/2):77–90.

HOLT, H. 1979. "An Existential View of Neurotic Conflicts." *Modern Psychotherapy* 5:1–7.

HORA, T. 1959. "Existential Group Therapy." *Journal of Psychotherapy* 17:83–91.

JAMISON, K., D. WELLISCH, AND R. PANAU. 1978. "Psychosocial Aspects of Mastectomy: The Woman's Perspective." *American Journal of Psychiatry* 135:432–436.

JARVIS, J. 1967. "Postmastectomy Breast Phantoms." *Journal of Nervous and Mental Diseases* 144:266–272.

KAUFMAN, E. AND V. G. MICHA. 1987. "Psychotherapy with the Good-Prognosis Cancer Patient." *Psychosomatics* 28(10):540–548.

KLAGSBRUN, S. 1983. "The Making of a Cancer Therapist." *Journal of Psychosocial Oncology* 1(4):138–147.

KLEIMAN, M., M. MANTELL, AND E. ALEXANDER. 1977. "RX for Social Death: The Cancer Patient as Counselor." *Community Mental Health Journal* 13:115–124.

KOWAL, S. 1955. "Emotions as a Cause of Cancer: 18th and 19th Century Contributions." *Psychoanalytic Review* 42:217–227.

KUEHN, P. 1986. *Breast Care Options*. South Windsor, CT: Newmark.

KUSHNER, R. 1975. *Breast Cancer: A Personal History and an Investigative Report*. New York: Harcourt Brace Jovanovich.

LEWIS, F. 1982. "Experienced Personal Control and Quality of Life in Late-Stage Cancer Patients." *Nursing Research* 31:113–119.

MAGUIRE, P. 1978. "Psychiatric Problems After Mastectomy." In P. C. Brand and P. A. van Keep, eds. *Breast Cancer: Psychosocial Aspects of Early Detection and Treatment*. Baltimore, MD: University Park Press.

MAGUIRE, P. 1976. "The Psychological and Social Sequelae of Mastectomy." In J. G. Howells, ed. *Modern Perspectives in Psychiatric Aspects of Surgery*. New York: Brunner-Mazell, pp. 76–89.

MAJES, M. L. AND G. A. MENDELSOHN, 1979. "Effects of Cancer on Patient's Lives: A Personological Approach." In G. C. Stones, S. Cohen, and N. E. Adler, eds. *Health Psychology*. San Francisco: Jossey-Bass, pp. 225–284.

MARRAM, G. 1978. *Group Approach in Nursing Practice*. St. Louis, MO: C. V. Mosby.

METZGER, L. F., T. F. ROGERS, AND L. J. BAUMAN. 1983. "Effects of Age and Marital Status on Emotional Distress After a Mastectomy." *Journal of Psychosocial Oncology* 1(3):17–33.

MEYEROWITZ, B. 1980. "Psychosocial Correlates of Breast Cancer and its Treatment." *Psychological Bulletin* 87:108–131.

MILTON, G. 1973. "Thoughts in the Mind of a Person with Cancer." *British Medical Journal* 4:221–223.

MORRIS, T., S. H. GREER, AND P. WHITE. 1979. "Psychological and Social Adjustment for Mastectomy." *Cancer* 40:2381–2387.

MORRIS, T., S.H. GREER, K.W. PETTINGALE, AND M. WATSON. 1981. "Patterns of Expression Anger and Their Psychological Correlates in Women with Breast Cancer." *Journal of Psychosomatic Research* 25:111–117.

MULLEN, H. AND M. ROSENBAUM. 1962. *Group Psychotherapy*. New York: Free Press.

OSTCHEGA, Y. AND J. JACOB. 1984. "Providing Safe Conduct: Helping Your Patient Cope with Cancer." *Nursing* 65:43–46.

OWENS, R. F., J. J. ASHCROFT, S. J. LEINSTER, AND P. D. SLADE. 1987. "Informal Decision Analysis with Breast Cancer Patients: An Aide to Psychological Preparation for Surgery." *Journal of Psychosocial Oncology* 5 (2):23–33.

PARSELL, S. AND E. TAGLIRENI. 1979. "Cancer Patients Help Each Other." *American Journal of Nursing* 74:650–651.

PECK, A. 1972. "Emotional Reactions to Having Cancer." *American Journal of Roentgenology and Radium Thermonuclear Medicine* 114:591–599.

PETTINGALE, J. W., M. WATSON, AND S. GREER. 1985. "The Validity of Emotional Control as a Trait in Breast Cancer Patients." *Journal of Psychosocial Oncology* 2(3/4):21–30.

RAY, C. 1978. "Adjustment to Mastectomy: The Psychological Impact of Disfigurement." In P. C. Brand and P. A. van Keep, eds. *Breast Cancer: Psychosocial Aspects of Early Detection and Treatment.* Baltimore, MD: University Park Press.

RAY, C., J. FISHER, AND T. K. WISNIEWSKI. 1986. "Surgeons' Attitudes Toward Breast Cancer, its Treatment, and Their Relationship with Patients." *Journal of Psychosocial Oncology* 4(1,2):33–43.

ROBBINS, G. 1973. "Nursing Management of Patients with Breast Tumors." In H. Behnke, ed. *Guidelines for Comprehensive Nursing Care in Cancer.* New York: Springer.

ROSS, P. 1976. "Psychological Problems in Surgery." *Resident and Staff Physician* 22:76–79.

SABO, D., J. BROWN, AND C. SMITH. 1986. "The Male Group and Mastectomy: Support Groups and Men's Adjustment." *Journal of Psychosocial Oncology* 4(1/2):19–31.

SARTRE, J. P. 1947. *Existentialism.* New York: Philosophical Library.

SCHAIN, W. 1976. "Psychosocial Impact of the Diagnosis of Breast Cancer on the Patient." *Frontiers of Radiation Therapy and Oncology* 11:68–69.

SHAFFER, J. AND M. GALINSKY. 1974. *Models of Group Therapy and Sensitivity Training.* Englewood Cliffs, NJ: Prentice-Hall.

SIMONTON, C. O., S. SIMONTON, AND S. CREIGHTON. 1978. *Getting Well Again.* Los Angeles: J. P. Tarcher.

SPIEGEL, D., D. R. BLOOM, AND I. YALOM. 1981. "Group Support for Patients with Metastatic Cancer: A Randomized Prospective Outcome Study." *Archives of General Psychiatry* 38:527–533.

SPIEGEL, D. AND M. C. GLAFKIDES. 1983. "Effects of Group Confrontation with Death and Dying." *International Journal of Group Psychotherapy* 33(4):433–447.

STEFANEK, M. E., L. P. DEROGATIS, AND A. SHAW. 1986. "Psychological Distress Among Oncology Outpatients." *Psychosomatics* 28(10):530–539.

VACHON, M. AND W. LKYALL. 1976. "Applying Psychological Techniques to Patients with Cancer." *Hospital and Community Psychiatry* 27:582–584.

WEISMAN, A. D. AND J. W. WORDEN. 1986. "The Emotional Impact of Recurring Cancer." *Journal of Psychosocial Oncology* 3:5–16.

WHEELER, J. AND B. CALDWELL. 1955. "Psychological Evaluation of Women with Cancer of the Breast and of the Cervix." *Psychosomatic Medicine* 17:256–258.

WHITAKER, D. AND M. LIEBERMAN. 1964. *Psychotherapy Through the Group Process.* New York: Atherton Press.

WITKIN, M. 1975. "Sex Therapy and Mastectomy." *Journal of Sex and Marital Therapy* 1:290–304.

YALOM, I. 1975. *The Theory and Practice of Group Psychotherapy.* New York: Basic Books.

YALOM, I. 1980. *Existential Psychotherapy.* New York: Basic Books.

16

Cancer Communication/Education on a Head and Neck Service

Andrew Blitzer, MD

What exactly is cancer education and how do we teach cancer care to students? Who is the teacher? A teacher is someone who imparts knowledge about a subject to others while continuing to acquire new knowledge. Teachers should be so enmeshed in their field that they eat it, think it, and dream it. They will be good teachers since they will impart some of their enthusiasm about the subject to the students. Clinical teachers instruct by example, so they must display excellent clinical skills to win the respect of their students. They must be thorough, competent, kind, and compassionate to win the respect and cooperation of their patients. The students will learn from their mentors, who are role models.

What is education? Mark Twain said that it is what is left when everything that has been learned has been forgotten. Since this concept of education in cancer care is ill-defined, it becomes much harder to decide how to impart this commodity to our students. Cancer care includes the medical technicalities of treating disease; the conflicts of the unknown; interpersonal relationships with the patient, family and friends; the coordination of the multidisciplinary team; and dealing with one's own emotions. Education in cancer care must of necessity include all of these areas. In the medical setting, emphasis is usually placed on the technical aspects of treatment; the psychosocial aspects may not even be mentioned. Not only mentioning, but coming to grips with the patient's fear and anger, his family, his financial problems, is of the utmost importance. Often concern in the psychosocial area will aid in the technical area by making

---

The author wishes to dedicate this essay to the loving memory of his mother, Lyrene Lave Blitzer.

patients willing and eager partners in their therapy. A good deal of this material can be formally taught, but much of it must be taught by example, if it is to have real meaning in the clinical setting.

The technical aspects of cancer care are often confusing to the student since there are so many controversies and uncertainties. In some medical centers, patients are staged and put on protocols. Often, this is done in an arbitrary and impersonal way, not including the patient in the decision. This is a mistake. The patients are already losing a lot, and they should not have to give up their dignity in addition. People are much more cooperative and respond much better when they are included in making decisions about their own destiny.

In other medical centers there are turf battles between the various groups of professionals who offer treatment for the patient's disease. Their contradictory statements and arguments are only confusing for the patients and for the students. Some of the best cancer care education can be delivered to students with a multidisciplinary tumor board, where all of the issues of a patient's care can be addressed by experts in many fields, including psychiatry, social work, nursing, nutrition, and others. In such a forum, the student is able to see the many facets of a patient, facets perhaps never before realized.

Surgeons, who must teach their house staffs to be the surgeons and teachers of the next generation, must be special people. The great surgeon/teachers will constantly challenge their students and bring them right to the edge of disaster, but not let them fail. This may well be beyond where they dreamed of going, but it is important for the student to feel both the joy of succeeding and the pain involved in accomplishing the goal. The great surgeon/teacher also learns from each of these encounters.

Cancer care teachers must bring out the best of each of their students' personal resources. Telling a patient he or she has cancer or is dying, speaking to the family, being honest with the patient, require great personal strength on the part of the care giver. Often, people will try to avoid the situation, or to make it someone else's duty. Nonmedical people do not understand the special nature of the doctor-patient relationship. They ask, "How can you stand working with the dying patients? It must be constantly depressing." They do not understand the joy of being able to help, even if only in a small way, a patient dying of cancer who is afraid, in pain, and in need of someone to trust and depend upon. This special relationship has to be taught to those who are afraid of becoming involved with the dying.

To further complicate this discussion, we, the teachers of cancer care, are also medical practitioners who are always learning to improve our own skills and abilities, as well as trying to contribute to our chosen fields. Therefore we are not only teachers, but students; our colleagues may also be both our teachers and our students.

To better understand this complex interaction, we can picture it graphically (Figure 1). We start with a surgeon-teacher. Arrows both lead to and radiate from the surgeon, denoting the intake as well as the transmission of knowledge. The surgeon has an impact on the many groups around him, the most obvious being the postgraduate students (residents) and undergraduate students who are assigned to the service. Much of the knowledge is transmitted in nonverbal communication, by role modelling. How we respond to a cancer patient not only becomes important to the doctor and the patient, but becomes a message to the students about how one should conduct oneself in this special relationship. We, as teachers, must not only carefully study and analyze what we say to our students, but spend time assessing our doctor-patient relationships to make sure we transmit the correct nonverbal messages as well. We learn a lot about this special relationship from *our* teachers—the patients. Patients will teach much about what they need, both physically and emotionally, if given the chance. Included within this special teaching relationship are the patients' family and friends, who often see things that we do not. They can be very helpful in informing us about aspects of the patient that are unfamiliar to us. They are often the harshest critics and the most vociferous fans. After processing this information intellectually, we can then transmit it to our students.

We, the surgeons, also continue to learn from our mentors. Usually the best teachers keep themselves available to speak to their students about difficult problems and continue to give their students advice and support as needed. The surgeon should also continue to innovate methods and techniques of evaluating, treating, and rehabilitating patients with cancer. The constant pursuit of improved cancer treatment and more humane management is the mark of all true practitioners. The surgeon-teacher should teach surgeons in other hospitals, and in other cities and countries by contributing to programs of local and national meetings as well as to journals.

Another most important interaction is between the surgeon and the rest of the cancer care team—including nurses, psychiatrists, social workers, and clergy—who also view the care and can teach the surgeon about their perspective on it. Their views allow the surgeon to see beyond the narrow confines of surgery. Often this continued open channel will allow the surgeon to find out information that neither the patients nor the family related to him. It also gives the surgeon a sounding board for making difficult decisions, by providing an avenue for the advice of others who understand the difficulty of the situation and the options available.

Another group that must enter this equation is the public, including the media, the legislators, and the people. Because of the significant cuts in government funding, and the outright discontinuation of many programs, the sick, poor, and old are receiving less than ever. For the good of our patients, we must make the public aware of what will happen to them and their families if the funding cuts are implemented in an attempt by government to "balance the budget." The public should know that programs that are seeking new treatments, assistance programs for cancer patients and their families, and hospice centers are being cut or eliminated. We must teach our legislators about cancer care, the problems of cancer patients, and why funding cuts may adversely affect cancer patients. This is perhaps the only way a government that is trying to find ways to save money can be forced to respond to the needs of these patients. Similarly, at a local level, we must teach administrators and people involved in HMOs what is necessary for good cancer care. These organizations are designed to be profitable, and not primarily or necessarily to consider quality of health care. Cancer care is special care and is often very expensive. Subscribers to HMOs must understand what they are getting and apply pressure to the organizations in order to receive the kind of care they need and want.

In short, the role of surgeon-teacher in cancer care is a very complex one. The educational process should be multifaceted with each participant learning from the other. The result of such a system would benefit all, including the patient who is receiving the care.

Figure 1. The Teaching Interaction.

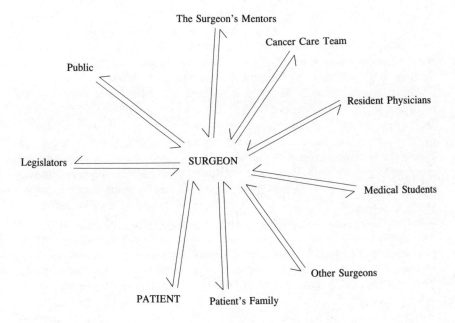

17

Caring for the Patient with Head and Neck Cancer

Mary Jo Dropkin, RN, MSN

The term "head and neck cancer" refers to a malignancy in the area that lies above the clavicle but excludes the brain, spinal cord, axial skeleton and vertebrae. The exact etiology of head and neck cancer remains unknown, but excluding skin lesions, the tumors are frequently found in conjunction with history of heavy smoking and alcohol intake. It is estimated that 40,800 cases of head and neck cancer occur each year in the United States, accounting for 14,600 deaths annually (American Cancer Society 1984). Although head and neck cancers comprise only a small percentage of all cancers, they warrant special attention owing to the drastic structural, functional, and psychosocial disturbances that can result from the disease and its treatment.

Although many lesions that arise in the area are amenable to detection and treatment in the early stages of disease, the anatomic complexity of this region frequently predisposes to aggressive tumor growth with subtle clinical manifestations. The current treatment of choice for most head and neck cancers is surgery in combination with radiotherapy. Chemotherapy is also being used more widely along with surgery or radiation in an effort to improve survival rates. A radical surgical approach, often necessitated by occult tumor location, poses unique problems, however, in relation to quality of survival. Ablative cancer surgery may necessitate removal of relatively large portions of bony and soft tissue from the face or neck to the extent that normal appearance is permanently altered. Structural loss in this region is also associated with functional loss such as aphonia, speech impairment, or difficulty swallowing. The resultant disfigurement and dysfunction create considerable emotional upheaval as defects in the head and neck area are particularly threatening to senses of identity and self-concept. Society's emphasis on physical attractiveness imposes an additional social burden upon the individual who sustains facial disfigurement or dysfunction after surgery. Within this context, complete recovery entails reintegration of the defect. This occurs as the patient gradually learns to compensate for anatomic alteration through optimal use of residual structure and function, maximal restoration of self-expression, and reestablishment of sociability (Dropkin 1981). The ultimate goal of the caregiver is to assist the patient through this process. It is essential, therefore, that the caregiver be aware of the significant impact he or she can have on this course, and of the behavioral manifestations of the patient's progress.

THE PATIENT

Frances MacGregor's work with the congenitally disfigured clearly indicates that one's worth as a person is frequently assessed according to facial characteristics (MacGregor 1967). Deviance from society's aesthetic expectations is often judged harshly or deemed socially unacceptable. Surgically acquired disfigurement/dysfunction includes a number of additional problems. The patient's perception of his or her own facial appearance and function has accumulated over a lifetime and is stored in memory. Structural or functional alteration in the head and neck region creates a distortion between the image stored in memory and the real appearance and functional ability after surgery (Scott 1983). A patient who undergoes total laryngectomy, for example, experiences two major bodily changes: creation of a permanent tracheostome in the neck (disfigurement) and aphonia (dysfunction). Memory traces of skin integrity and the sound of one's own voice conflict with the postoperative reality. In addition to anxiety, which accompanies awareness of bodily alteration, the patient must undergo the grief process. According to the perceived physiologic and psychosocial value of the structure or function, the patient needs to mourn each loss. The postoperative patient may also experience tremendous fear of rejection or abandonment by others because of the alterations in appearance. The most significant component of the impact of surgically acquired disfigurement/dysfunction ultimately seems to lie within a social context, or the concern with others' reactions.

THE CAREGIVER

Others' reactions to surgically acquired defects in the head and neck area were recently described by the development of the Disfigurement/Dysfunction Scale (Dropkin et al. 1983). This scale evolved from an attempt to quantify the relative severity of impact of disfigurement/dysfunction upon the patient by using others' reactions to typical postoperative defects. The sample consisted of 100 registered nurses in a large urban cancer center. The high degree of agreement within this sample indicates that consensus exists on the impact of each type of disfigurement and dysfunction upon the patient as well as upon the caretaker. It also raises questions concerning the possible influence of caregivers' perceptions upon their interactions with patients.

It is not unusual for the caregiver to experience some anxiety when first seeing severely disfigured patients. The visual impact can be quite disconcerting. This anxiety is thought to arise from the subconscious fear that a similar occurrence could happen to the viewer (Masson 1963). With this particular population, the caregiver cannot use the defense of depersonalization, or detachment of operative site from the patient. This region represents identity to both patient and caregiver. Reactions to dysfunction, on the other hand, may be somewhat less intense. Dysfunction is generally related to the ongoing personal manner in which self has been presented throughout life, rather than to sudden change in facial appearance, a criterion more dependent on social convention. The perceived reaction of the caregiver is highly meaningful however, as he or she is usually one of the first people to observe the patient's altered appearance or self-presentation. Technical competence, evidence of compassion, and simple face-to-face interaction can all serve to reassure patients that they will not be rejected because of the way they look, and that their identity has not been irreparably altered.

COPING

The Disfigurement/Dysfunction Scale has been used in a study designed to describe behavioral manifestations of coping after major head and neck sugery. Specific self-care and resocialization behaviors were identified which reflect the impact sugery has had on the patient and thus on his residual capacity to cope (Dropkin and Scott 1983). Three basic principles underlie the coping process (Donovan and Pierce 1976). Some interesting parallels may be seen between patient and caregiver interaction.

Self-care following head and neck surgery usually requires touching the area and viewing it in a mirror. Tactile and visual limits are set in this manner which eventually help to "confine" the defect. Rather than perceiving the defect as overwhelming to his identity, the patient can ultimately see it as a relatively small aspect of his anatomy or of the total person. Important tasks to facilitate gradual incorporation of the stoma following total laryngectomy, for example, include self-suctioning and cleansing of the skin around the area.

The second method utilized to cope with disfigurement and dysfunction involves emphasis on self or the person rather than physical characteristics, and should be inherent in all patient/caregiver interaction. In this way, anxiety related to bodily alteration can be reduced over time and attention can be redirected to self as the essence of continued life. For example, following total laryngectomy and prior to alternative voice rehabilitation, the patient must communicate in writing. This is often difficult and frustrating for the patient as well as time-consuming for both patient and caregiver. Taking the time to sit with patients and encourage them in dialogue, however, lets them know that whatever they want to communicate is equally important to you, regardless of the form it must take.

Finally, the ability to view physical limitations as other than liabilities can help in coping with postoperative deficit. If any form of alternative voice following total laryngectomy, for example, is compared to normal speech, it will be perceived as a liability. If viewed, however, within the context of diagnosis, surgery, and rehabilitation, the production of any form of alternative speech can be considered a great asset.

There may be a long interval between the initial surgery, or acute phase, and the terminal phase of cancer. During this time the patient must somehow be able to live with the defect(s). It is important, therefore, to identify the patients who do not appear to be coping adequately according to recently established postoperative "norms" (Dropkin and Scott 1983). These patients will likely need more specific and intensive assistance with the reintegration process. Reports in the literature indicate that inability to cope with surgically acquired disfigurement/dysfunction leads to the development of chronic problems such as increasing anxiety (Owens 1968), depression and social reclusiveness (Nordlicht 1979), or noncompliance with post-discharge care (Bryce 1981). Each of these maladaptive behaviors can represent a serious threat to the quality of remaining life.

Further research is needed in this area to determine whether short-term coping predicts long-term coping. Anecdotal observation indicates that adequate coping with disfigurement/dysfunction during hospitalization enhances reintegration after discharge and may ultimately facilitate responsiveness to intervention during the terminal phase of illness.

The following case history is that of a caregiver who has worked with the head-and-neck cancer patient population for the past 10 years. It is a personal account of one patient's course as perceived by a nurse who cared for him from the time of his initial surgery to his death approximately one year later. It describes the evolution of this caregiver/patient bond with particular emphasis on feelings generated in the caregiver during the patient's terminal phase. It illustrates the difficulties as well as the rewards of caregiver commitment, the power of nonverbal communication, and responsiveness to nurturing.

CASE HISTORY

Ted was admitted to the hospital again last December. He had suddenly developed massive (parastomal) recurrence in his neck and shoulder and he was in great pain. He was admitted for radium implantation and pain management. He was angry . . . and so was I.

Ted had his total laryngectomy a little over a year ago. He used the Blom-Singer voice prosthesis to speak and ultimately did really well with it—so well, in fact, that Ted was the one I'd call when I wanted to demonstrate this form of alternative voice to patients who had undergone a similar procedure. It was always so rewarding to see him and to observe how he'd work with the patients. He was always able to instill so much hope in them. He was bright and good-looking and impeccably dressed, but, most of all, so full of life and warmth. It's hard to believe that he'd once had a terribly difficult time coping with his own laryngectomy. It's easy to forget that his pathology report at the time of surgery showed highly infiltrative aggressive disease.

Ted had wanted so much to be home for Christmas. So, once his pain was manageable with oral medication, he was discharged. Ted was very aware of his situation, asked lots of questions, and quickly became adept at the new self-care tasks he now needed to know—how to maintain his shrinking airway and how to care for the skin in the area of tumor growth. He was back to writing again at that point—the prosthesis had to be removed because of tumor encroachment on the trachea. He told me that he'd had a "good life" and that he was "not afraid to die," but was *very* much afraid of any more pain. His sister was going to come into town to take care of him until "the end." I promised to stay in close touch and, meanwhile, he was to receive chemotherapy as an outpatient.

He never did make it to the outpatient department. I called chemotherapy the day of his appointment to let them know that he had, instead, been readmitted to the hospital. That was in the beginning of January—he'd become terribly weak and depressed and seemed to have aged several years in less than two weeks.

I remember taking one look at him and saying "I'm glad you're here now." He nodded in agreement. I didn't bother to ask what happened with his sister—she wasn't there. I did hope, however, that at least his close friend would continue to be as supportive to Ted as he'd been since the time of his surgery. He seemed to leave the hospital awfully fast that day, though—Ted was barely settled into his room. Ted was so weak he could hardly write, so we "talked" for just a little while about how miserable he was feeling. I told him I'd do everything I could to make him comfortable and so before I left for the day I brought him all the things I knew he'd need—pain medication, paper, pans, extra blankets, ice water and his favorite, apple juice!

I was off the next day and then was sick with the flu for several more. I was worried about Ted, but kept reminding myself that although we'd always had very special nurse–patient "chemistry," he'd be in good hands in my absence. Nevertheless, when one of the staff called to see how I was doing, I asked her to please tell Ted I had the flu and would be back as soon as possible—just in case he might have been feeling lonely or abandoned. I wasn't able to return to work until two days prior to a scheduled trip to California for five days. By now, Ted was counting on a chemotherapy treatment he was to receive. He told me that he was frightened by the rapidly enlarging tumor—and he hadn't even seen it. I was horrified to see the huge fungating mass that had developed on his neck. And I was frightened too—afraid he'd have a horrible death by carotid artery hemorrhage and that I wouldn't even be there to ease the terror of that kind of death. I had no control over that, though.

The morning I left for California, I went to see Ted first thing as usual, and there he was sitting in a wheelchair staring at the breakfast tray in front of him. It hadn't really occurred to me that he was too weak to feed himself until, as I was talking, I just happened to pick up his cereal bowl and started stirring. He opened his mouth . . . and I fed him the entire bowl. Later that morning, before I left, I was letting his staff nurse know that he'd now need help feeding himself, and I started to cry. In addition to the tremendous sadness I felt over the prospect of losing Ted, I felt guilty about having to leave him (on a vacation, no less)—about not being able to be with him when he needed someone more than ever—especially now that I knew his family and friends weren't going to be there for him.

When I said good-bye to Ted, I gave him the usual big kiss and big bear hug and a spontaneous, "I love you lots," to which he smiled and responded, "You, too." He told me to have fun and I thanked him and told him I'd be back in a few days. I didn't know if I'd ever see him again. It was so frustrating, too, because I felt we still had a lot of "unfinished business" between us. I thought that as we had worked together on his grief and then had coped with laryngectomy, we could work together on making his last days as comfortable as possible. I was hoping to help him work through his depression and progress into acceptance—if we could only have a little more time. As a friend said before I left though, "Maybe he'll wait for you." I hoped he would.

While I was in California, I tried to keep my thoughts of Ted under control. It hurt so much already—anticipating his loss. I realized that if he was still there when I got back, I should rest and relax as much as possible now because I would need all my strength then. Sometimes, when I'd wonder if I had enough strength to deal with this, I'd think to myself, "Well, you don't *have* to do this." I knew the most difficult part for me was going to be letting him go. So how could I watch Ted die a little more each day and still be therapeutic—help him to let go? Well, if the therapy was also in the energy and the care and the feeling, then I'd continue to do my best to see him through.

It broke my heart to read Ted's chart when I got back. He had spent the week in continuous depression, agonizing pain, and had had a series of tests that revealed bowel, liver, and bone metastases. It was as if his whole body had just "exploded" with cancer. He was no longer eating by mouth, his neck was filled with fungating, necrotic tumor, and he had developed a large bedsore on his back—it hurt him so much to lie on either side, he would constantly reposition himself on his back when the nurses would leave. He refused further chemotherapy, telling the doctor he wanted to "die in peace." Thank God he was on morphine "drip" (IV) by then, which was finally beginning to alleviate the tremendous increase in his pain. I noticed two small vases of flowers in his room and a little stuffed teddy bear holding a big red satin heart on his bedside table. I was so glad somebody had thought of him, even if that person couldn't stay with him. I could understand, but it made me so angry. . . .

Ted was unable to write at all by this time. He slept a good deal, but was easily aroused. I was shocked when I saw him, despite what I'd just read in the chart. He opened his eyes and formed the words, "You're back!" with his mouth. He'd always teased me about my cold hands, but this time he just closed his eyes and smiled as I gently stroked his forehead. From that point, everything I did for him was done with great gentleness—more than I knew I had—from my tone of voice to wetting his lips and mouth with a little apple juice. Each day after that I would assist the staff in caring for Ted, with his bath, back care, and bed linen change. Each day (with one exception) I'd make myself leave at the usual time, knowing how important it was for my own stamina to do that. Each day I'd let him know when I was leaving, when I'd be back, and the names of the other nurses taking care of him. We'd give our usual kiss and bear hug—gentle ones now, but always reaffirming our affection of each other. One day I told him that it was hard for me to leave him, but that if I didn't leave for a while each day I wouldn't be any good to him when I was there. He nodded in understanding but kept looking at me—I'd come to know his facial expressions so well by then. My eyes filled with tears—some even fell on him as I was bending over his bed. He looked surprised and then very concerned. I told him that it just made me awfully sad to see him going through all this. He gave me the gentleness that time—his face told me, "It's not really as bad as you think" . . . and I felt better.

One morning the night nurse told me that Ted seemed to be very angry at times during the night and also very frightened. I knew he was frightened of being alone and fortunately my case load was light that week so I spent the day with him and stayed several hours later that night. I didn't see any anger or fear, but I did see the terrible spasms of pain he was having again—all the more poignant beause he was unable to cry out. His morphine requirement tripled that day and I refused to leave until I knew he was comfortable.

Besides physical care, what did I do with Ted all that time during those last two weeks? What did I say? I'd hold his hand and stroke his forehead—sometimes for hours. All I'd usually say very softly was that I was there, that I was going to stay with him that he was in a safe place where nothing would harm him. There was so much more I wanted to say—like how much I was going to miss him, how I would always cherish the unique and special relationship we were sharing, and that the increased awareness, sensitivity, and gentleness that I was gaining would remain with me always; it would become a part of me. I didn't say any of it at that point, though. I was sure there were many thoughts he wanted to share with me, too, but he wasn't able to speak or to write, so neither did I. During bedside care, Ted would try so hard to stay awake as much as possible. It became increasingly difficult for him to keep his eyes open for any length of time, but it was as if he didn't want to sleep as long as there was life. After that I'd sit either on his bed or right next to it to give him as much contact as possible. He'd keep opening his eyes and once he was able to focus, would just look at me, and I at him, and there we'd sit quietly and contentedly just looking into each other's faces. I realized even then that those were some of the most beautiful and meaningful moments I'd ever spent with another human being. Eventually, he wouldn't be able to fight the sleepiness anymore and he'd drift off peacefully. I'd always stay for long periods after that, and would always be sure he was pain-free and had that peaceful expression before I'd leave.

The day before Ted died, he began to experience increasing periods of apnea—up to 30 seconds each minute. His pulmonary secretions increased profusely, his pulse weakened considerably and grew increasingly irregular, and his urine output almost stopped completely. I didn't think he was going to wake up at all that day, so when he open his eyes for a short time I remembered telling him how glad I was to see him after he'd been sleeping so long. He was too weak to smile back but his eyes did, and then with some effort, he said my name before drifting back to sleep. I left his room for only one brief period that day, during which I just sat and cried as I was eating my lunch. The staff was wonderfully supportive. Just before I went back to Ted's room, I suddenly felt this incredible sense of peace that seemed to come out of nowhere—acceptance, at last! I knew that I was finally ready to let him go. Once again I left the hospital that afternoon assuming that I would never see him again, but this time the intense emotions I'd felt those last weeks seemed more resolved.

The next morning I felt a kind of urgency about getting to work. Strange, because I knew intellectually that it was highly unlikely Ted would still be there. Well, he was—looking worse than ever and essentially unresponsive, but pain-free and peaceful. When the staff nurse came in to take care of him I helped her bathe him, shave him, give him back care and change his sheets. As usual I told him softly that we'd have to turn him from side to side to change his bed, but that we would do so very slowly and gently and that I would watch his face carefully for any sign of discomfort. At one point when I was holding him toward me, he scrunched up his face for an instant, seemed to yawn and then smiled! As we slowly turned him on his back, I explained that we would gently roll him over the bump of sheets in the middle of the bed and that we'd finish the bed change as quickly as possible in case he was experiencing any discomfort. As I was furiously smoothing out the sheet underneath him, the nurse to whom he was turned noted that his apnea seemed even more prolonged than it had been. We turned him gently on his back again and observed him closely for several minutes—he was dead. I don't know whether his last breath was while he was literally in my arms, but I do know that it was effortless and that he was at peace, free of pain and surrounded by love.

That was only three weeks ago. I think of Ted often and I miss him alot. But my feelings of loss are increasingly overcome by an incredible sense of fulfillment—as I remember all the extraordinary things we shared and how much we were able to give to each other. And besides all that, I now have this little stuffed teddy bear sitting right on my desk—holding a big red satin heart.

REFERENCES

AMERICAN CANCER SOCIETY. 1984. *Cancer Facts and Figures.* New York: American Cancer Society, Inc.

BRYCE, D. 1981. "Unique Features of Head and Neck Malignancies Which Relate to Their Management." *Journal of Otolaryngology* 1:3–9.

DONOVAN, M. AND S. PIERCE. 1976. *Cancer Care Nursing.* New York: Appleton-Century Crofts.

DROPKIN, M. J. 1981. "Changes in Body Image Associated with Head and Neck Cancer." In L. Marino, Ed. *Cancer Nursing.* St. Louis: C. V. Mosby Co.

DROPKIN, M. J. ET AL. 1983. "Scaling of Disfigurement and Dysfunction in Postoperative Head and Neck Patients." *Head and Neck Surgery* 6:559–570.

DROPKIN, M. J. AND D. W. SCOTT. 1983. "Image Reintegration and Coping Effectiveness after Head and Neck Surgery." *The Journal, Official Publication of the Society of Otorhinolaryngology and Head and Neck Nurses* 2:7–16.

MACGREGOR, F. C. 1967. "Psychosocial Approach to Patients with Facial Disfigurement." In D. Woods-Smith and P. Porowski, eds. *Nursing Care of Plastic Surgery Patients.* St. Louis: C. V. Mosby Co.

MASSON, R. L. 1963. "An Investigation of the Relationship Between Body Image and Attitudes Expressed Toward Visibly Disabled Persons." Unpublished doctoral dissertation, New York University of Buffalo.

NORDLICHT, S. 1979. "Facial Disfigurement and Psychiatric Sequelae." *New York State Journal of Medicine* 9:1382–1384.

OWENS, N. 1968. "A Study of Personality Changes in Males with Severe Facial Deformity During the First Six Months of Adjustment After Radical Surgery for Cancer.'' Unpublished doctoral dissertation, New York University.

SCOTT, D. W. 1983. "Quality of Life Following the Diagnosis of Breast Cancer.'' *Topics in Clinical Nursing* 4:20–37.

18

The Role of the Head and Neck Tumor Board in Clinical Cancer Education

Peter A. Shapiro, MD

Patients with head and neck cancer frequently are disfigured by their illness or its treatment, and in general have a rather guarded prognosis. These factors create a psychological burden not only on the patients, but also on their caretakers. In working with the Head and Neck Service at Columbia-Presbyterian Medical Center for a number of years, I have been impressed that this burden is borne more lightly by more senior attending physicians than by the resident staff, and I have wondered why this should be. What aspect of training enables the head and neck surgeon to deal with his work in so calm and resolute a manner? Observation of the weekly meetings of the departmental Tumor Board has led me to the conclusion that this meeting does more than teach information about cancer and its treatment. In addition, it conveys a way of being and feeling as a physician which is extremely adaptive for those who would work in this difficult field. How this is done and what is conveyed is the subject of this chapter.

The Head and Neck Tumor Board meets Wednesdays at 11:00 A.M. in the room between the ward and the clinic. At the front of the room is a small chair for the patient. Facing this are several rows of chairs, and on the side of the room are a couch and some armchairs, which seem to be reserved for the professors. In this setting, patients from the inpatient ward and the clinic are discussed in order to review their diagnosis and make plans for treatment. In attendance are the head and neck surgeons, an ENT resident or two, a radiotherapy attending and residents, an oncologist, an oral surgery attending and residents, a dentist concerned with prosthetic devices and rehabilitation, a speech therapist or two, and sometimes the unit head nurse. The patients wait in an anteroom. Their cases are presented, they are invited in and examined briefly, and they are sent out to wait again, to speak to the resident after the conclusion of the rounds.

The Tumor Board is a social structure designed to carry out certain functions, and while its manifest function is to develop treatment plans for patients, it also serves other purposes, by means of its particular organization. The structure of Tumor Board creates a particular type of educational experience; it teaches a way of thinking about cancer and its treatment. Inculcating this way of thinking is as important an educational goal as the transmission of information about particular cases or particular diseases. It is the music that counts as much as the words.

By the term "structure" I mean the set of expectations and rules by which Tumor Board operates. It is precisely the existence of these rules that distinguishes the Tumor Board from any other meeting of staff at which a patient's case might be discussed, including lunch in the doctors' cafeteria or chats in the hall or locker room. What, then, are these rules, the formal characteristics which define Tumor Board?

TUMOR BOARD PROTOCOL

The first rule, and *sine qua non,* is the rule to have rules. Tumor Board has a definite protocol. When protocol is not observed,—for example, if attendance is poor or the starting time is delayed—morale suffers, and protocol is quickly reinforced.

Case Presentation. Tumor Board meetings begin with the resident's case presentation, which is brief and focuses on the lesion. A common feature of the presentation is the remark that no old chart is available and that the patient is not well known to the resident. For residents there is little continuity of patient care; they rotate through different hospitals, the clinic, the ward service, and so forth.

The patient is invited in, seated, possibly asked a question or two by the attendings present, and examined in a limited fashion. Usually this examination is quick and silent, but on occasion leads to further questioning and checking. There may be some preliminary discussion of the staging of the lesion, its location, and so on, while the exam is proceeding. The patient rarely says a word except when spoken to.

Opinions. The resident is asked to formulate the case and his or her proposed treatment and other options. The attending head and neck surgeon then reviews the diagnosis and staging, cites other cases and relevant literature, and critiques the resident's formulation or preparation of the presentation. The surgeon makes a treatment recommendation, and then turns to the radiotherapist and asks for his or her opinion regarding the use of radiotherapy in this case. The radiotherapist cites statistics for staging, radioresistance, and survival, and concludes with his or her recommendation. Then the oncologist comments on chemotherapy, protocols, staging, and survival vis-a-vis the particular patient. The oral surgeon, psychiatrist, or prosthodontist may add their comments. The residents may then question, reformulate, and raise hypothetical questions, with which the attendings must deal.

Entertaining Alternatives. Even in cases for which the diagnosis dictates a particular treatment in a particularly clearcut manner, one of the constant and remarkable features of Tumor Board is the effort to entertain alternatives. Chemotherapy and radiotherapy are always mentioned, even when surgery is expected to be curative as a sole modality of treatment, and surgery is always discussed even for advanced and unresectable disease. This is described as "possibly palliative" or "the only hope of a cure." Even when radiotherapy is expected to be 100 percent curative, the statistics on surgical treatment are cited.

Nonconsideration of Nonmedical Viewpoints. One might say that nonmedical viewpoints are excluded from Tumor Board, but this would be a bit unfair. Somehow these views never come up. The psychiatrist has found it difficult to make constructive comments about aspects of the patient and his problems in Tumor Board. The speech therapists are silent, the family's experience of caring for the patient is not discussed, his social role is never considered. Reference may be made to the patient's smoking or drinking as a source of poor outcome or a compliance issue, often with a kind of challenge to the psychiatrist to do something about these behaviors. The psychiatrist, knowing that it is unusual that he or she can do anything about them in patients not inclined to change, and that those so inclined often do so without intervention, remains silent.

There is occasional acknowledgment of the disfiguring effect of a proposed surgical treatment, but the topic quickly turns to techniques of reconstruction.

I do not mean to be criticizing the staff in this property of the Tumor Board's work, only describing its functioning. The medical staff is not insensitive to these issues in their patients' care, but deal with them outside of Tumor Board. They tend to do so on an individual, not communal, basis, and without the same systematized approach. In Tumor Board, however, the emphasis is on accurate diagnosis and staging, proper work-up, percentage survival and other statistics. For this reason, Tumor Board can at times seem boring. The medical students do not seem to like it. They sit in the back of the room, cannot see or understand the examinations, and daydream during the discussions. There are other reasons for their behavior as well, or course.

Agreement on a Plan. The final rules of Tumor Board which I would like to mention are these: the participants in the discussion agree to agree on a plan, and they agree to follow it through to the end. The plan is followed through.

There is no changing horses in the middle of the stream. This does not mean that the staff is inflexible and not adaptable to the changing needs of the patient, but rather that, apart from emergencies, it is determined in advance at what point it will be appropriate to consider a revision in the plan.

For example, a patient with cancer of the larynx and a large metastatic mass in the right neck was seen in Tumor Board. The decision was made to perform a laryngectomy, followed by radiotherapy to reduce the tumor mass in the neck, and then to proceed to radical neck dissection. However, after radiotherapy was complete, the neck mass had completely disappeared. This patient was presented again to Tumor Board: Perhaps the plan to proceed to neck dissection should be abandoned? The response in the Tumor Board, ultimately, was that in fact the very representation of the patient for consideration was inappropriate; the plan had to be carried through, and only then should the patient return to decide on the next step. The attending—whose comment was, "Of course, with a mass like that we always do the neck, because microscopic disease might remain after radiotherapy, but in this case I just thought maybe we could wait"—was hooted down by his senior colleagues.

And this leads to the final rule of Tumor Board: that there are penalties for violating the rules—mainly, criticism and shaming—and even attendings are not immune.

THE LESSONS OF TUMOR BOARD

My aim has been to lay out the formal rules which define the Tumor Board, for the purpose of describing its role in cancer education—not as a place where information is transmitted but as a place where professionals in various stages of training are subjected to a particular form of professional socialization, taught a way of thinking and being in relation to cancer patients, in order to better be able to provide treatment. What are the lessons that Tumor Board teaches?

The first lesson is use of obsessiveness and isolation of affect to combat anxiety. The resident must present both succinctly and thoroughly. Each attending in turn restates the case. It is repetitively labeled, categorized, and classified. The patients presented may have terminal disease, ulcerations, bleeding. They may have neglected their care for months, to the point that once-curable disease has now become incurable, but all of this is only noted in the same cool, clinical tone. When the residents become too strident or insistent, too heated in the discussion, the attendings silence them. When they stay cool, the discussion may be extended. This dispassionateness may be exciting and attractive to students, but may also be off-putting, depending on the degree to which the students identify with the patient instead of striving to identify with the staff.

In the same vein, personal feelings of hopelessness and depression are not allowed. What is talked about is the concrete plan of action—what can be done, not what can't. Incurability is acknowledged, but even remote chances are pursued—grasping at straws, even when what is proposed is awful to contemplate. What is stressed is adherence to the proper way of going about treatment, not outcome.

Marcus (1983) has described the professionalization experience of medical students as one in which adherence to the rules of the craft is instilled as a substitute for a primitive idealism that requires good outcome as its sole criterion of success. This substitution is achieved by shaming for deviation from professional norms of conduct, and is necessary in order that physicians not be demoralized in the course of treating fatal or incurable disease. Tumor Board exemplifies the idea of adherence to craft norms; following a process properly becomes the standard of judgment of performance in place of outcome. Failure to follow the process, as in the case of the attending mentioned above, leads to shaming. This is to the good, as head and neck cancer patients, as a whole, have a poor prognosis.

Third, Tumor Board teaches routinization. Although the individual case is considered, it is considered chiefly to determine its type. The case is a specimen of a type; the type dictates the treatment. The use of routinization has been described (McIntosh 1977) as an aid for staff and patient coping with cancer, especially the management of doubt and uncertainty.

Fourth, learning to think in accordance with the rules of the Tumor Board helps to protect against the deleterious effects of denial. That is, the plan is carried through, and adherence to this rule keeps the staff from short-cutting the treatment with the hope that a partial treatment is enough. In the example cited above, the disappearance of the visible tumor after a course of radiotherapy led the attending to contemplate avoiding a radical neck dissection. On confrontation, though, he knew that microscopic disease could well remain. The plan, as he himself noted, is made because sometimes we "forget" our line of reasoning in the heat of the moment.

Finally, the Tumor Board process protects against anxiety. Kucharski and Groves (1976-7) have described a situation in which staff request psychiatric consultation for a patient they see as withdrawn, depressed, or hostile. The patient is one who has suffered mutilation or disfigurement but is not found by the psychiatrist to meet the staff's description. In essence, these consultations are called for because the patient's mutilation stirs fantasies of aggression in the staff, which are anxiety-provoking. Recently a staff nurse described her experience caring for a patient who had had a hemimandibulectomy for recurrent cancer. The lower left quarter of the patient's face had been removed, and a flap to fill in the gigantic defect had become necrotic, leaving the oral cavity uncovered. The nurse said that when, after a day at work, she sat across the dinner table from her mother, she saw not her mother's face but the mutilated head of her patient—an intrusive, recurrent image which was extremely disturbing. This case, however, is a rarity on the Head and Neck Service, despite the common occurrence of mutilation. The staff have a plan, they know to do, and they are not afraid.

In summary, Tumor Board, through its defining formal characteristics, teaches the management of affect in the care of cancer patients, and aids in the development and maintenance of professional identity.

REFERENCES

KUCHARSKI, A. AND J. E. GROVES. 1976–77. "The So-Called Inappropriate Psychiatric Consultation Request on a Medical or Surgical Ward." *International Journal of Psychiatry in Medicine.* 7(3): 209–19.

MARCUS, E. 1983. "The Role of Liaison Psychiatry in the Clinical Training of Medical Students: A Psychoanalytic Approach". In J. B. Finkel, ed. *Consultation-Liaison Psychiatry: Current Trends and New Perspectives.* New York: Grune and Stratton, pp. 267–284.

MCINTOSH, J. 1977. *Communication and Awareness in a Cancer Ward.* New York: Prodist.

19

Colon Cancer: A Prototype for Consideration of Psychosocial Aspects of Care

Frederick Herter, MD

Colon or rectal cancer is a prototypical cancer type and thus provides a good model for a discussion of the psychosocial aspects of clinical cancer education. We know a great deal about it, our methods of treatment are reasonably well established, and we know the course of the disease well. Unlike many cancers, however, it has very few variables in its behavior patterns; it is predictable.

It has been widely reported that colon cancer is regarded as one of the major cancers with environmental causes rivaling lung cancer. It is certainly related in one way or another to what we eat or what we don't eat. Its geographical distribution points quite clearly to environment as the initial carcinogen. Its incidence remains relatively constant in males and females.

FACTORS AFFECTING PROGNOSIS

Most cancers of the colon begin with a preexisting abnormality in the mucosa of the colon. We know, within reasonable bounds, how long it takes for a clinical cancer to develop. The disease spreads in a predictable way. Initially, very few cancers of the colon and rectum metastasize by way of the bloodstream. Most of them exhibit a pattern of spreading or invading the lymphatic channels and thereby entering the lymphatic pool in the abdomen, specifically, in the mesentery of the bowels where groups of lymph nodes reside.

The prognosis for colon and rectal cancer can be determined by a number of different criteria. Size is one of them. This seems logical; there is a linear relationship between the size of the tumor and the anticipated incidence of lymph node metastasis, so that a one-centimeter tumor of the colon will not, just from its size alone, produce metastasis in any person, whereas a seven-centimeter tumor will produce metastasis in perhaps 75 percent of all those afflicted. There is one exception; if the tumor gets bigger than seven centimeters, a reverse trend exists; it may be that such a tumor is biologically different from small tumors in terms of the immune factors, or it may be that the invasive properties of the tumor itself allow it to grow to a large size without producing fatal metastasis in the interim. Therefore, the largest tumors of the colon and rectum are apt to be the most curable. This is an interesting phenomenon which also holds true for cancers of other sorts.

Differentiation—what cells look like under the microscope—is extremely important in terms of prognosis, although only 5–10 percent of these tumors are truly anaplastic, with undifferentiated cells. Those particular to that subset of cases have an extremely ominous prognosis. The vast majority, 90 percent or more, are either well or moderately well differentiated, creating a big gray zone. The anaplastic tumors, however, regardless of treatment, regardless of what we do with them, are killers.

The depth of invasion of the tumors is another important factor with a bearing on prognosis. Does the tumor go through the bowel wall? Does it invade the surrounding perirectal tissue? By far the most reliable index of prognosis is whether or not the lymph nodes are involved, how many are involved, and where the involved nodes are located.

The relationship of lymph nodes to prognosis has been well established in breast cancer. We have the same type of information for colon cancer: for example if one lymph node is involved and if that lymph node is close to the primary tumor, it has very little relationship to prognosis. If more than one lymph node is involved, anticipated survival in that individual is much decreased. There is a great difference between one and two nodes, but where they are located is also important. Obviously, a central node afflicted by a tumor shadows a bad and a quick ending, whereas involvement of a node close to the tumor does not.

Colon cancer is one of those cancers for which an operation can be performed without having made a tissue diagnosis. Why? Because when cancer occurs in the colon, the X-ray picture is classical and one can make diagnosis without any equivocation. On the basis of the radiographic evidence alone, it is common to submit patients for major operations without corroboration by tissue diagnosis . The X-ray diagnosis may be substantiated with the colonoscopic examination and a direct biopsy, but, in most instances, this is not necessary.

Involvement of the lymph node and differentiation of the tumor are the two most important factors in establishing a prognosis. Upon the return of the laboratory report, roughly two weeks after the operation, the surgeon has a clear idea as to whether the patient is cured or doomed. These predictions are obviously not infallible; there are exceptions. These issues are raised simply because colon cancer, in contrast to many other types of cancers, including breast cancer, has a highly predictable behavior. If there are a number of nodes involved, and particularly if they are far away from the tumor, the outlook is grim indeed.

In terms of nonsurgical treatment, high energy X-ray therapy and chemotherapy are both used preoperatively or postoperatively in large cancers of the rectum. Radiation therapy is a valuable adjunct in treatment of rectal cancer, but not for that of the colon. Chemotherapy is relatively ineffective.

When the pathology report indicates that five nodes are involved, two in the intermediate group and three in the central group—signs of a very severe prognosis—the temptation is to say, ''Let's do something else and let's do it right now.'' The evidence of the benefit of adjunctive chemotherapy in such cases is, however, not encouraging, so the surgeon and the patient have a difficult decision to make. The temptation is to become aggressive, but the facts say that here, treatment really does not influence the overall survival figures or the disease-free period after the operation.

Chemotherapy, by and large, is reserved for the patient who comes back with a symptomatic recurrence, one that is producing pain, or one with an obstruction. Virtually all recurrences make their appearance within the first two years, unlike other cancers. If the disease is going to kill the individual, it does so within the first five years. Here is one cancer in which survival can be predicted with great accuracy. Only about three percent of patients who will die of this disease die after the fifth year. Indeed, on the fifth anniversary of the operation the patient can come come back to the doctor and say, ''I've brought a bottle of champagne, let's celebrate!''

Metastases that kill are generally those that invade the liver. Because they go directly to the growth part of the splenic circulation, and because that circulation goes through the portal system and through the liver first, metastatic tumor cells are often trapped in the liver rather than in other parts of the body. Eventually, death from cancer of the colon occurs, in most instances, because of liver involvement. Some metastases in the liver and even in the lung are resectable, encouraging hopes for cure. Hence, we can never truly shut the door on a patient with a demonstrated recurrence or a metastasis until we examine that option very carefully. There are a number of patients with a single metastasis or with a few metastases in the liver, restricted to one lobe or the other, who are alive and well many years after resection of that particular lobe. Likewise, patients who have produced solitary metastasis in the lung have been cured by lung resection.

When a recurrence does occur in the liver that is impossible to treat in terms of curative surgery, the patient may still live a long time, and this is one of the unhappy aspects of this disease. The average survival for a patient with minimal but inoperable metastatic disease of the liver is about eleven months. If half the liver is gone, survival is obviously going to be shorter. Once in a while, a patient will live for two or three years with metastatic disease in the liver, suffering a slow attrition, a weakening, loss of appetite, loss of weight, loss of energy, and in some cases discomfort or pain, which may vary in degree.

PSYCHOSOCIAL ASPECTS

As in all cancers, there are a number of critical factors in the evolution of colon cancer that have profound psychosocial effects on the patient. These bear examination in terms of inclusion in the professional curriculum. The first is the impact of the diagnosis on the patient. Second is the nature of the cancer itself, and whether, by its very nature and by the necessary treatment, it will destroy something fundamental in the function or self-image of the patient. In the case of colon cancer, the individual is relatively fortunate. Resection of the bowel and anastomosis of the bowel ends can restore normal bowel function. The patient experiences no loss of body image, sustaining only a scar on the abdomen. Cancer of the rectum presents a different challenge to the physician, because the sphincter mechanism, which is responsible for continence, must be destroyed if the operation is going to be curative. That means the patient must face a colostomy, which entails a great psychic trauma. Moreover, especially if the patient is young, there is imminent danger of total or partial loss of sexual function. These two fairly drastic changes have to be faced both by the patient and by the doctor caring for him or her. It is the responsibility of the health care team to counsel the patient and to help arrange for further counseling.

The third critical time occurs when the pathology report arrives and the doctor must analyze the tumor and determine the importance of the node involvement. An accurate prognosis has to be made for the patient. If there is ambiguity and the doctors must play a waiting game, not knowing whether a recurrence may happen, there is a problem in terms of candor: Should the doctor tell the patient, "We don't know what's going to happen to you. You've got a node involved. We have no therapy for that." Should the doctor convey that ambiguity to the patient if in fact the patient may already have been cured?

If the doctor is following a patient and finds that the cancer has returned, then there is another crisis in management.

Finally, it should be kept in mind that the period of attrition that precedes death is apt to be longer in patients who have this disease than for patients with many other types of cancer, so that the patient and family will therefore require considerable psychosocial care that includes the physician as active participant.

20

The Cancer Patient
with Alzheimer's Disease

Mary Anne Zubler, MD

Care of the patient with Alzheimer's disease who develops carcinoma was at one time a relatively simple matter; the two diseases were simply not considered together. Patients with cancer were treated according to their usual treatment, and this applied to patients with Alzheimer's disease as well. However, the emphasis on quality of life has brought into sharp focus the philosophical and ethical issues that surround care of such patients.

It is not uncommon for an oncologist working in a VA hospital to see, once or twice a week, a patient with a chronic dementia—one who has been cared for at home or in a nursing home—who has been brought to the hospital with an abnormality on chest X-ray that is regarded as cancer until proven otherwise. (In the public hospitals, we constantly struggle with the fact that many of our patients are unknown to us prior to their appearance at the door in a debilitated state, and therefore, we do not have the advantage of a prior long-term relationship with them. However, for many physicians working in the community, a relationship with the patient and his or her family has been long established, and some idea of the patient's wishes may often be construed.) In treating such a patient, quality-of-life proponents would have us consider what quality of life remains to the person. But we must first consider what quality of life is.

Quality of life has been described in terms of present life styles, past experience, hopes for the future, dreams, and ambitions. When a person's hopes are matched and fulfilled by experience, it can be said that the quality of life is good. It is obvious from this definition that quality of life in these terms is only applied with difficulty to patients with Alzheimer's. In the end stages of Alzheimer's, in fact, patients do not show signs of having ambitions or hope for the future. It is obvious that the incompetent patient (i.e., one afflicted with advanced Alzheimer's disease) cannot communicate to us what could make them happy and what life-prolonging treatments they would rather refuse, either for the sake of more comfort in their last days or for the sake of shortening the last days or weeks of an increasingly confining dying process. Likewise, the physician is handicapped by the fact that he cannot explain to the patient either the treatment or the testing procedures, and thus perhaps communicate to the patient that the benefit to be obtained from sometimes uncomfortable treatments or testing is worth the discomfort. In caring for these patients, medical and nursing personnel are frustrated at times, in part because the way in which they assess their own competence and personal worth is reflected by how well they care for their patients, as judged by the patients' response to their ministrations. In cancer patients, medical treatment may not be the curative treatment that one would hope, but one can offer support to help the patient through the deeply emotional process of dying. With the Alzheimer's patients one is deprived of such personally satisfying experiences.

The quality of life has certain characteristics: it fluctuates with time, it is modified by age and experience, and it may be expressed in terms of satisfaction, contentment, happiness, fulfillment, and the ability to cope. Some of these terms may indeed be applied to patients with Alzheimer's disease, since such qualities can, albeit in a primitive way, be measured. While one may not be able to determine the presence of happiness in these patients, a measure of satisfaction or contentment may be observable.

How then are we to make the decisions concerning these patients? Are we simply to relegate all of them to a "no-treatment" group? Obviously not, simply because there are some stages of Alzheimer's in which patients are more able to communicate their wishes concerning their disease to their physician. Whenever possible, patients should be involved in decision making. However, when a patient receives a diagnosis of Alzheimer's, it is usually past the point at which he or she may participate meaningfully in any decisions about further medical care. How then might we make decisions for these patients? Two principles may apply. The first is *the principle of substituted judgment,* in which one is guided to make the same decisions the patient would have made if the patient were capable of doing so. We can often surmise what this might be on the basis of past experiences with the patient and/or the family's experiences with the patient. We assume that most patients will approach death and decisions regarding it in the same way they approached life and the decisions they faced earlier. Some patients with Alzheimer's, therefore, have given us an idea of what might be their approach to the difficult situations that they encounter in the process of dying. However, many patients do not realize the magnitude of the situations they will encounter in dealing with cancer, and the discomforts and emotional problems that may overwhelm them during this time. As caretakers of such patients, we often invoke another principle for making such decisions, *the principle of best interest,* in which we try to act to promote the patient's presumed best interests.

One can see that these two principles may be at odds in a particular patient. We may feel that it is not worthwhile to continue the patient's life in the manner in which we see him or her existing, but the patient may have made some previous statement or had a previous approach to life that would indicate that he wanted to live at all costs. (One sometimes wonders if people understand what the phrase "all costs" means.) It is observed that the principle of best interest is probably used more often in treating patients with Alzheimer's, because we cannot communicate with them to determine anything about their own judgment concerning decisions during this time.

Also hampering us considerably in making decisions "in the patient's best interest" is the dilemma that the patient's best interests are reflected through our own eyes, and therefore of necessity are our own best interests. That is, we project onto these patients, the quality of life we see as appropriate and therefore quality of life in these situations is based on highly generalizable and personal assumptions. For example, we assume that most people would prefer to avoid pain and to live longer. However, if these assumptions are both correct, we run into problems because these preferences can and do conflict—for example, when longer life can be had only at the cost of expensive, highly invasive, or painful therapy.

In most patients with Alzheimer's, treatment generally is conservative and based only on relief of any symptoms the patient might have. Upon initial contemplation, this seems to be a reasonable thing to do for these patients. However, many competent patients, when given the same alternatives, will opt for chemotherapy or other types of therapy and a possible remission of their cancer. Why should not the same be done for patients with Alzheimer's disease? On the other hand, why should patients be forcibly treated with difficult therapy without their understanding—treated only that they may live for a short time, with no appreciation (that we can determine) of that time as "best"? Clearly there are no easy answers to these questions. Some believe that until medicine and the law collaborate to develop best-interest standards, the terminal patient who cannot indicate his or her wishes will usually be treated according to the quality-of-life projections of the attending physician, in conjunction with the family, and subject only to the availability of resources.

It has been said that the emphasis in the provision of health care to the demented should be on maintaining functional capabilities. Is this an appropriate way to approach these patients? If so, we must then define functional capability. We all know of people who are living in the community with early stages of

Alzheimer's disease, who, despite their limitations, are able to survive without an overwhelming amount of support. Usually there are groups such as Visiting Nurse Associations, church and synagogue associations, caring neighbors, and concerned relatives who give these patients what they need to fill the gaps in their own ability to survive. If such patients develop cancer, it seems reasonable to attempt to achieve a remission and relieve symptoms, with the hope of returning them to their former, if minimal, functional capacity. However, a patient who is dependent on assistance to bathe, dress, eat, and transfer from bed to chair; has no idea of person, place or time; and/or spends most of the time in bed, may be seen as a patient whose quality of life is minimal at best and who should not be treated. However, given a broader definition of quality of life, this patient may still have some satisfaction and contentment in his minimal existence and therefore, should be treated as a competent patient.

It may be proposed that in caring for patients with Alzheimer's disease who develop cancer, these steps should be followed in order to most ethically approach them:

1. The problems and priorities must be defined at the outset: What is the patient's basic problem in terms of his or her symptom complex, or life-threatening problems? What are the priorities by which we rank each of these problems? Will the most important problem be control of pain or treatment of a reversible disease process, in order to return a patient to his or her prior functional state?

2. Any form of intervention must be tailored to the individual patient. Obviously this means that, if the patient has any ability to contribute to the decision, he should be encouraged to do so, and the patient's functional status should be taken into account when determining treatment interventions. Those patients who are most debilitated and most close to death from Alzheimer's disease may continue along a relatively contented life style if the cancer can be brought under control.

3. Evaluation of the result of the intervention is essential. Once one has embarked upon a treatment plan, it is important to continually monitor it to see whether or not it is reaching the objectives that have been set out. If the patient is suffering more from the effects of the treatment than the disease, it may be appropriate then to change the course of action.

Caring for patients with Alzheimer's, particularly those who develop cancer, will never be an easy problem, and we have a special responsibility to steer a course between either resisting premature requests from weary relatives or staff to stop all life-prolonging efforts, or else applying overzealous efforts up to the last breath of life. Because life is a moral requisite of community, and because relatives and friends do not want to be seen as abandoning a loved one, situations in which health professionals are uncertain about what is best should be resolved in favor of extending life where possible. This same policy should apply where friends or relatives strongly urge it, since they will have to live with these decisions long after the health professionals have transferred their attention to other patients. The right to life is equally a right for all human beings, and by itself, incompetence should not diminish that right.

In any event, as Dyck (1982) points out:

> "People of good will are bound to differ when it comes to caring for terminally ill, incompetent patients. Without a strong consensus for curtailing life-sustaining efforts, impartiality demands that their lives be supported in principle. At the same time, impartiality demands that the comfort of the patient's last days be considered in circumstances where competent dying patients would sometimes put that first. A consensus of all parties appropriately concerned with the care of such patients should be reached, so that life is not taken in the face of the inevitable frustrations of caring for severely demented dying patients. Hopefully the future will bring us something better to offer those with Alzeheimer's and other mentally debilitating incurable diseases."

REFERENCES

DYCK, A. J. 1982. "Ethical Aspects for the Dying Incompetent." 1982. *Journal of the American Geriatrics Society* 32(9):661–664.

ADDITIONAL READING

LO, B. AND L. DORNBRAND. 1984. "Guiding the Hand that Feeds: Caring for the Demented Elderly." *The New England Journal of Medicine* 311(6):402–404.

ROWE, J. W. 1985. "Health Care of the Elderly." *The New England Journal of Medicine* 312(13):827–835.

SCHNEIDER, E. L. AND J. D. REED. 1985. "Life Extension." *The New England Journal of Medicine* 312(18):1159–1168.

SCHNEIDERMAN, L. J. AND J. D. ARRAS. 1985. "Counseling Patients to Counsel Physicians on Future Care in the Event of Patient Incompetence." *Annals of Internal Medicine* 102:693–698.

21

The Impact of Group Counseling on the Terminally Ill

Calvin E. Selfridge, BA, MA

Cancer is a particularly terrifying illness for so many reasons; pain, discomfort, wasting (cachexia), and probable disfigurement. There is *no* certainty about cancer except the probability of recurrence and, ultimately, death. It is perhaps the fear of living with the unknowns of cancer that cause the greatest terrors in the patients. Death may be a certainty for them, but what happens until it occurs can terrorize them. Thus, the terminal cancer patient experiences denial, pent-up anger, guilt, helplessness, being out of control, curtailment of the future, goals left unattained, hopes abandoned, and threats to self-esteem through an increasing dependence on the hospital staff as physical degeneration proceeds. The terminal cancer patient struggles with living and dying in an atmosphere of tension and crisis.

At issue for me as a counselor is how to enable the terminal cancer patient to develop coping abilities. Primary among these would be alleviating loneliness and isolation, managing anxiety, maintaining self-esteem, mobilizing hope, increasing warmth of communication, and establishing trusting relationships.

My work with terminal cancer patients at Calvary Hospital in the Bronx has focused on developing one-to-one relationships with each patient I counsel. This focus has had many positive results, but it has also spurred my thinking about group counseling for the terminal cancer patient. Often I have heard patients express feelings, thoughts, hopes, and beliefs which I felt could be of great benefit to other patients who were dying. Yet I was also very aware of the limitations that most patients placed upon themselves, expressing a sense of worthlessness and an unwillingness to associate with other sick people, especially those sicker than they. Such attitudes would seem to be a hindrance to establishing a group counseling process for terminal cancer patients, whose habitual behavior patterns since hospitalization have been withdrawal, avoidance, and inconsistent awareness of dying. But my belief that each of the dying patients whom I have met has something to share with other patients is stronger than their fear that they have nothing left to give and that existence during their last days is meaningless. I am also aware that the patients' capacity to resolve their terminal crises will be strongly influenced by the extent and quality of communication that occurs during the group process. This awareness demands that as a counselor, I have the training and skill required to tolerate close contact with dying and death; that I come to terms with my own fears and anxieties concerning my mortality; and that I have the ability to share in the suffering, conflict, and anguish of the terminal cancer patient.

If there is one purpose in establishing a terminal cancer counseling group, it is to enable the patients to live psychologically fulfilling lives up to, and including, the moment of death. Terminal cancer patients need people in their lives who are willing to communicate with them about their concerns and fears. A counseling group can enable patients to express, clarify, and specify the daily difficulties involved with dying. Such issues as loneliness, grief, loss, fear, depression, anxiety, pain, nausea, and bodily incapacitation could be explored during group sessions. Each patient-member faces similar physical and emotional problems, and each member could help other members to deal with these problems. Supportive group therapy could be effective in enabling the terminal cancer patient to obtain emotional support and coping skills from other group members. This sharing of coping skills helps to establish meaningful daily goals as well as maintaining self-esteem and self-image. The patient may come to realize that he or she does have much to contribute, even in the face of dying and death.

In the establishment of this particular terminal group, one criterion is of primary importance: only those patients who have no external support group— no family, friends, or relatives—will be invited to participate. This limitation is established simply because many of the patients at Calvary Hospital are in this category and, as a result, are in greater danger of experiencing isolation and a sense of abandonment. Consequently, these patients may benefit most from becoming involved in a counseling group that would allow them the freedom to express and share their feelings and relieve the sense of "aloneness" in facing death.

Other criteria used to screen group members are as follows:

(1) A diagnosis of terminal status and an estimated survival time of 3-6 months;
(2) An acceptance of terminal status by the patient, i.e., the patient is not in a state of massive denial;

(3) The client must be an inpatient and have been referred by the staff at Calvary Hospital;

(4) Factors such as age, stage of illness, socioeconomic status, cultural background, professional status, and religious affiliation should be considered when establishing group membership. It would seem better, for example, to group patients who are closer in age and life experiences as well as stage of illness, while cultural backgrounds, and professional status may have less effect on the development of the group.

It would also be my intention to maintain the traditional psychotherapeutic group; one that is relatively closed and whose members meet on a regular and consistent basis. Even though other researchers such as Rickett and Koffmann have strongly endorsed the open-group approach because of the nature of cancer and its treatment, I feel strongly drawn towards a closed-group environment because of the group cohesion and sense of trust generated in such a setting. Also, on a more practical note, many of the patients at Calvary Hospital are over age 70 and suffering from periods when their memory is affected by age rather than their cancers. The sense of continuity and consistency in group membership will be less likely to add to the already disrupted memories of the patients.

An ideal group size for this terminal cancer group would be five to seven patients. They would meet for a period of six weeks. Given a diagnosed period of survival of three to six months, a six-week group process would have a strong chance of continuation with a minimal loss of membership.

GOALS

Realistic group goals for terminal cancer patients ought to be set by the patients, who know best what their needs and wants are at this critical point in their lives. My role would be as a facilitator in helping them to attain as many of the realistic goals that have been set as possible.

When the patient becomes a group member, the loneliness, isolation, and need for withdrawal that result from the pain of guilt, anger, and helplessness are greatly diminished. Courage gathered from the thoughts and experiences of other group members helps the patient to face difficult conflicts, abandon ineffective defenses, and gain insight into coping with approaching death. Participation in such a group also encourages the patient to vent feelings of fear, anxiety, shame, and dependency. Sharing and greater tolerance develop as the patient becomes more secure in this new and supportive environment.

But what is the critical role of the group? In my opinion, it is to help each group member focus on living fully in the face of death. Such a role can be met in the following ways:

(1) Enable the group to determine patterns and meanings in each member's life and support the development of each member's full potential as an individual;

(2) Encourage the patient to examine his or her values, priorities, and sense of meaning in life;

(3) Support the efforts of each member as he or she works through "unfinished business";

(4) Focus on development of a sense of autonomy and the ability to meet the external demands of dying.

There is no doubt that dying is a traumatic experience, yet there is a component to it that must be worked through if acceptance is to be achieved. To this end, the group will examine the process part by part, and by doing so begin to cope better with each part. Out of this process a definite cohesiveness can emerge which will enhance the courage of all who remain with each other until the end.

GROUP PROCESS

Work in a group process environment involves a most important factor, the discomfort of those patients on a terminal trajectory. In my brief experience at Calvary Hospital, many uncomfortable situations have arisen, causing me anxiety, nervousness, and frustration. Although group sessions are likely to intensify this discomfort, I believe they should not be minimized or avoided.

Often, what a terminal patient chooses to discuss or share with the group will be only the easiest issues for them to confront. Therefore, body language and what is *not* said will acquire a deeper significance. Much communication is "shadowed" and the group leader must be aware of cues. Death and dying will most definitely be discussed, although they may be addressed in veiled terms. Such attention to cues is a critical issue and touches on facilitating the process of settling "unfinished business."

Yalom and Speigel (1981, p. 234) state that group therapy allows for the formation of several "curative" factors:

(1) *Universality*. A sense of all group members being in the same situation, and a gradual diminishment of the sense of being singled out (Why me?);

(2) *Altruism.* A sense of helping oneself by helping others. The client experiences an enhanced sense of interpersonal confidence and self-worth through helping others;

(3) *Instillation of hope.* A sense that others have moved past problems involved in dying;

(4) *Cohesiveness.* An unconditional acceptance and belonging, which offsets the dreadful isolation often experienced by the dying. The group becomes the focal point in patients' lives and they no longer feel isolated from the rest of humanity.

When the patient in a group decides what problems will be discussed and when discussions will occur; when the group is non-directive, non-confrontational, informal and supportive, then I believe that direct and honest communication about cancer and the course of his or her dying can be voluntarily shared.

Feelings of anger; rage; fears of loss of control, dependency, and death, are all in need of expression by group members. The environment described above can provide innumerable possibilities for interaction and learning as group members come to feel less passive and less victimized, and become adept at living in the here and now. Time is so fleeting for them—too precious to be wasted on trivial matters—and so personal growth is accelerated and a deep sense of purpose in life begins to form. Interestingly, the group comes to understand that they have a purpose *because* they are dying. Group members are encouraged in their understanding that they can teach others what they had learned about life as a result of their encounter with death; how to face death openly and accept loss. This sense of purpose alone can make death more meaningful.

As a facilitator, I would seek to help group members develop more effective ways of dealing with the dying process; perhaps, most directly, maintenance of some control over that process. By encouraging a heightened assertiveness, full partnership in decision-making, and a valuing of their own time and energy, facilitation would help each patient to focus on living as richly as possible. Through exposure to other terminally ill members of the group, patients are helped to face their common problem, and to approach death in an environment that promotes self-respect, support, and love. Death, therefore, becomes the final stage of growth.

The possibility that some group members will die during the course of the group is to be expected. It is reasonable to question what the effect will be of those deaths on the group morale; obviously, members will become acutely aware of their own vulnerability because of the death(s) of a group member, and they will experience grief reactions to those losses.

Each patient needs time and guidance to cope with approaching death; differences in each patient's stage of illness affects the the group. There is no question that acute physical deterioration and death of a group member will threaten group cohesiveness. But when such deaths occur, the group must be encouraged to feel the sadness, pain, and anguish fully. For it often happens that mourning is not only for the deceased but also for the group member who realizes that parts of his or her own life are slipping away. It is my hope that a group member's death will convey to the remaining members a sense "that the way one dies is significant and that even the last moments of life carry within them important choices." (Yalom and Speigel 1981, p. 238)

RESISTANCE

Three kinds of fear can inhibit the type of therapy I am proposing: those of the counselor; those of the client; those that arise out of the process.

The Counselor's Fears. For any counselor attracted to working in the field of death and dying, it is imperative that the personal issues of death be honestly and directly confronted. The counselor must recognize his or her own anguish and anxiety surrounding death and dying. Once these issues are laid bare, the counselor will be in a better position to empathize honestly with the existential pain and suffering his or her clients are experiencing.

Certainly, initiating a group counseling process with terminally ill patients can raise more fears and anxieties for the counselor. Primary among these may be a fear that the patients could be harmed psychologically through association with others who are terminally ill. A frightening and potentially dangerous possibility of opening a Pandora's box of emotions that might be very difficult to control must be taken into consideration. What *does* the counselor do with the raw emotions that are bound to erupt?

The Clients' Fears. The patients also have their own anxieties and fears— quite apart from approaching death—in participating in a group counseling process. Many of the counselor's fears and apprehensions may be shared by the client: issues of exposing raw emotions. Yet other fears are unique to the patients' position in life.

Most terminal cancer patients that I have met at Calvary Hospital have an expressed disinclination to associate with other patients that are ill, especially with those sicker than they. I've noticed in this regard a certain distancing and isolation. Dying, after all, is a task that must be done alone and often drains the physical and psychological energies of the patient. Perhaps it is this realization that makes the patients seek isolation; fear of further unnecessary drains on their energy.

I have also sensed that as the dying process accelerates, patients tend to withdraw, severing most social ties with the exception of one individual, with whom a bond is maintained until the end. The terminal patient may fear being unable to commit himself or herself to the group process because of a stronger need to withdraw in death.

Fears Arising from the Group Process. For the counselor and most assuredly for group members, the strongest fear generated in a group situation surrounds the death of a member. How does the group respond when a member dies? How does the group maximize the learning experience of each member as he or she confronts the process of dying and death?

To join a group process where the only bond is death and dying requires courage and the capacity for taking risks. The terminally ill person has an intense need to be seen as an individual; becoming involved in a group process could be perceived as a threatening loss of individuality unless the patient is helped to understand how needed and important his or her presence and experiences are as an expression of what is most individual about him or her: living and dying.

CONCLUSION

Because this chapter addresses questions and issues in the realm of theory and hypothesis, it is impossible to evaluate here the effects of the group process method of psychotherapy with terminal cancer patients. Yet those indications of success described in the literature indicate that such a process can enjoy a modicum of dynamic growth and development.

One striking fact that I encountered in pursuing my research, and which seems to indicate a definite bias against the terminally ill within the health service arena, is the extent to which psychological needs are ignored in terminal care. My experience has indicated that the dying have boundless needs to share and relate with other people. They want to talk about their hopes, dreams, fantasies, successes, failures, and what they are experiencing as they die. All too often they are denied this and allowed to die, alone, in an institution.

It is my belief that group counseling with the terminal cancer patient will prove that the dying person wants to talk, that one can talk with them, and that such efforts are meaningful and rewarding for all members of such a process.

REFERENCES

BOHART, J.B. 1979. "Group Counseling and Death Anxiety." *Death Education* 2: 381–390.

FRANZINO, M.A., J.J. GEREN, G.L. MEIMAN. 1976. "Group Discussion Among the Terminally Ill." *The International Journal of Group Psychotherapy* 26 (1): 43–48.

GARFIELD, C.A., AND R.O. CLARK. 1978. "The Shanti Project: a Community Model." *Death Education* 1 (1): 397–409.

GOLDBERG, F. 1984. "Personal Observations of a Therapist with a Life Threatening Illness." *The International Journal of Group Psychotherapy* 34 (2): 289–297.

HYLAND, J.M., H. PRUYSER, E. NOVOTNY AND L. COYNE. 1984. "The Impact of the Death of a

Group Member in a Group of Cancer Patients.'' *The International Journal of Group Psychotherapy* 34 (4): 617–627.

JACKSON, E. 1978. "Counseling the Dying.'' *Death Education* 1(1): 27–41.

KELLY, A.P. 1979. "Group Approaches for Cancer Patients; Establishing a Group.'' *American Journal of Nursing* 5: 914–915.

LESSER, I.M., AND I.D. GODOFSKY. 1983. "Group Treatment for the Chronic Patients: Educational and Supervisory Aspects.'' *The International Journal of Group Psychotherapy* 33 (3): 535–547.

LINDEMANN, E. 1979. *Beyond Grief: Studies in Crisis Intervention.* New York: Jason Aronson, Inc.

LINDENBERG, S.P. 1983. *Group Psychotherapy for People who are Terminally Ill.* Springfield, Ill.: Charles Thomas, Publishers.

SPIEGEL, D. AND M.C. GLAFKIDES. 1983. "The Effects of Group Confrontation with Death and Dying.'' *The International Journal of Group Psychotherapy* 33 (4): 433–449.

SPEIGEL, D. AND I. YALOM. 1981. "Group Support for Patients with Metastatic Cancer: A Randomized Prospective Outcome.'' *Archives of General Psychiatry* 38.

WHITMAN, H. AND G. GUSTAFSON. 1979. "Group Approaches for Cancer Patients: Leaders and Members.'' *American Journal of Nursing* 5: 910–913.

YALOM, I. 1977. "Group Therapy with the Terminally Ill.'' *American Journal of Psychiatry* 134: 396–400.

YALOM, I. AND D. SPEIGEL. 1978. "A Support Group for Dying Patients.'' *The International Journal of Group Psychotherapy* 28 (2): 233–247.

22

Adapting Time-limited Therapy to the Care of Persons with Cancer

Marilyn M. Rawnsley, DNSc

All science is the search for hidden likenesses . . . the progress of science is the discovery at each step of a new order which gives unity to what long seemed unlike.''

—Jacob Bronowski

The need for theory-based, cost-effective strategies that provide psychosocial support is essential to the notion of comprehensive health care for persons with cancer. Advances in biomedical science and technology have altered the prognosis of the disease in a majority of cases from that of an inevitably painful, debilitating decline toward death to one characterized by intensive surgical and medical interventions, dramatic, hopeful remissions, and all too often, discouraging, invasive recurrences.

Although most persons with cancer, despite the remissions and the apparent treatment successes, eventually die of the disease or its sequelae—including the complications of what Lewis Thomas (1974) has termed "half-way technology"—in general, a diagnosis of cancer no longer delivers a notice of impending death. Nevertheless, cancer still carries warnings of hard times ahead, of increased physical and emotional vulnerability, of underlying uncertainty about one's relations with others, and of threats to one's sense of personal control.

Cancer means unwanted change, and unwanted change involves real and anticipated losses on all levels of ego-investment. Examples of threatened losses include, but are not limited to, separation from familiar activities and surroundings, changes in appearance and energy, decreased ability to function independently, and the fear of rejection and abandonment by others. Anxiety about these unwanted changes contributes to, and is compounded by, a heightened existential awareness of just how tenuous one's claim on life really is.

In short, the same scientific progress which offers remedies for the physiological consequences of cancer, introduces problems in the management of the psychosocial dimensions of the disease. The unwanted changes that accompany the experience of cancer constitute a potential psychological crisis, in that customary ways of dealing with stress may not be adequate for the new challenges imposed by the illness and its implications.

The purpose of this essay is to describe the theoretical development and clinical application of a model I have designed to help patients strengthen their resources for dealing with the crisis of cancer. The theoretical framework of this model is derived from three sources: the substantive base of time-limited psychotherapy as postulated by James Mann (1973,1982), the concept of a "facilitating environment" as described by Donald Winnicott (1965), and the four standards of health as delineated by Judith Smith (1983): (1) clinical, (2) role-performance, (3) adaptive, and(4) the eudamonistic or holistic model (see Table-1).

TABLE 1
Theoretical Framework of Loss Therapy
(Rawnsley, 1986)

Assessment	Method	Goal
Construct: Universal conflict situations[1]	Construct: "Facilitating Environment"[2]	Construct: Standards of Health[3]
A) Activity vs. passivity	A) Brief psychotherapy-private practice model	A) Clinical—signs and symptoms of disease
B) Adequate or diminished self-esteem	B) Therapeutic Milieu—General practice settings	B) Role-performance—expressive and instrumental roles
C) Unresolved or delayed grief		C) Adaptive—Creative problem-solving
D) Independence vs. dependence		D) Eudamonistic—self actualizing, or holistic
Purpose:		
To identify characteristic pattern of response to loss as basis for therapeutic plan	To provide predictable professional support that fosters independence and motion towards health[3]	To expand evaluation of health and healthy behavior to encourage growth through loss

References:
1. Mann (1973, 1982) 2. Winnicott (1965) 3. Smith (1983)

From these theoretical sources I have derived a model for brief psychotherapy for persons with recurrent cancer. The propositions of Mann regarding universal behavioral responses to the prototypical loss experience of separation anxiety constitute the substantive base of the model. The role of the therapist is conceptualized within the context of Winnicott's writings on the influence of the "nurturing other" in encouraging independence. The outcomes of therapy are evaluated according to the standards of health explained by Smith as representing ideal composites of definitions and values from ancient Greek philosophy to modern thought. Since the theoretical derivation of the private-practice model has been reported elsewhere in the literature (Rawnsley 1982), the major focus of this chapter is to describe the process of adapting the principles of brief psychotherapy in caring for persons with cancer in general clinical settings.

The decision to investigate time-limited therapy as an appropriate modality for persons with cancer was reached after several years of working as a psychiatric consultant to nursing and social work staff in general hospital oncology units, outpatient oncology clinics, and community hospice services. In addition, my experience in collaborative practice with a clinical psychologist stimulated curiosity about the special needs of persons with cancer.

Examination of this rich clinical data-base revealed disquieting themes. Persons with cancer had ever-increasing options for chemotherapeutic, radiological, and surgical innovations aimed at aggressive attack on alien cell proliferation, yet there was little corresponding advance in the approaches to help persons maintain control over their life while they endured assaults to their physical being and alterations in their accustomed life style. As one client stated, "I think that the doctors are so busy congratulating me on how well my tumor is shrinking that they can't see how scared I am and how sick the treatments make me." Or, to quote another, "I guess I should be grateful that they have these drugs to try out on me, but instead I'm mad as hell at everyone, especially myself."

Patients admitted resentment, families expressed frustration, and staff were alternately confused or defensive. It seemed that biomedical technology had outdistanced human resources.

Discussions with, and observations of, other professionals strengthened the growing concern that our well-meaning interventions were not being effectively translated into techniques that encouraged patients to maintain control over their lives. Too frequently, the afflicted person's anxious plea for safety—"do whatever you think best"—was mistaken by professionals for healthy compliance. Too frequently, the uncomfortable or frightening feelings engendered in encounters with these clients interfered with professional ability to assess emotional responses within established frameworks of knowledge.

Patients were stigmatized as "cancer victims," with all the helplessness implied in the term.

Accordingly, in order to maintain the boundary that would identify us as separate from them, perhaps even to ward off a similar fate, or perhaps because so little is certain about its etiology, elaborate hypotheses were constructed about the emotional handicaps that precipitated or predisposed one to developing cancer. Often, such speculations and their derived therapies simply served the function of victim-blaming, further dividing the sick from the well.

From the dual perspective of psychotherapist with individual clients and psychiatric consultant for oncology staff (who were willing to risk personal involvement in the hope of learning more about their patient's emotional needs) qualitative data from therapy sessions was compared to patient–staff interactions. The purpose of this comparison was to address the basic research question, "what is happening here?" A major outcome of this joint venture was that the label "cancer victims" was discarded and patients were appreciated as human beings, just like us, who happened to be experiencing the crisis of cancer. And quite predictably, just like us, these patients were behaving in this dilemma the same ways they had behaved in the past. In other words, we were able to look beyond our biases and see that the illness *per se* did not totally account for a person's emotional response. Instead, the phenomenon being observed was an individual's characteristic pattern of managing stress. The stress, common to all these persons, was identified as unwanted change, i.e., the anxiety of real and anticipated loss that accompanies a life-threatening illness.

Therefore, psychosocial support of persons with cancer could be logically derived from a conceptual framework that allowed for an interpretation of individual behavioral responses to the universal human experience of loss. The substantive base of time-limited psychotherapy provided an explanation of loss and an approach to its resolution that could be appropriately adapted for the care of persons with cancer.

The substantive base of time-limited psychotherapy is derived from Mann's (1973) proposition that there are four universal conflict situations that express "all the ways that humans experience loss" (p. 27). These theoretical constructs are described as: (1) activity versus passivity; (2) adequate versus diminished self-esteem; (3) unresolved or delayed grief; and (4) dependence versus independence. They are rooted in the developmental perspective of object relations theory. These universal conflict situations are postulated to explain the behavioral responses that attempt to resolve ambivalence felt during the normal maturational crisis of separation individuation. Separation and loss are recurring life themes, and threats to sense of mastery or control of self in relation to the external world emerge whenever maturational or situational crises occur.

Since the experience of cancer can be considered a situational crisis, the behavioral responses to the actual and anticipated losses that accompany the condition can be said to be characteristic of an individual's pattern of resolving the ambivalence—reducing the anxiety—of separation-individuation.

For example, persons who ordinarily confront unwanted change with cognitive problem-solving approaches and a confident, assertive attitude, can be expected to take an active role in their treatment. Persons who characteristically use passive avoidance techniques that temporarily reduce anxiety but do not address the underlying issues will be more likely to demonstrate continued denial, displacement of anger, social withdrawal, and other affective responses.

All illness involves some increased dependence on others. For persons who have progressed on what Winnicott (1965) describes as the journey from dependence to independence—have achieved an ability to balance self-reliance versus reliance on others—increased dependency is a major threat to personal integrity. For those persons with a strong need to be taken care of by others, regression towards the absolute dependency of infancy—in which the external world is perceived as having all the power to fulfill or deprive basic needs— may present seductive illusions of security. In any case, the demands of the illness and its treatments will elicit reactions to dependency that need to be addressed.

New loss resurrects old grief. The familiar painful feelings must be acknowledged if mourning is to accomplish its task of divesting energy from lost objects. But feelings have no focus. Unharnessed by cognitive structure, they attach to old memories, to shadows from the past. Earlier losses that were not fully mourned intensify the difficulty in working through the immediate issue, and the significance of the actual or potential disruption is magnified by symbolic distortion from unresolved or delayed grief.

Those who have come through other life crises with continued or renewed self-worth and value will approach the trials of this illness, at least initially, with faith in their ability to conquer it. Those already beset by self-doubt and blame will demonstrate lack of confidence that their behavior can affect outcomes. Since self-esteem will be sorely tested during this experience, it is important to evaluate the patient's perception of how previous challenges were handled.

Of course, assessment in all dimensions of universal conflicts is fundamental to explaining and predicting behavioral patterns of response during the experience of cancer. The plan for psychotherapeutic support is contingent upon systematic identification of individual patterns of response to loss. Space does not permit elaboration of the interview technique that elicits information about past and present behaviors and the identification of the predominant conflict. In general, however, the method is conversational and open-ended rather than structured. Questions such as "Tell me about another time in your life when things seemed difficult . . . what did you do?" (coping), or "If you could change some things in your past, what would you change? " (loss) or "Talk about yourself as if you were describing someone I've never met" (self-esteem) are more enlightening than fixed questionnaires. Since such an open approach requires skilled interviewers, training and supervision must be available to staff.

Although individual assessment of the conflict pattern is the basis for the focus of the plan, some general principles derived from Smith's (1983) models of health can be considered. When people are newly diagnosed or are experiencing exacerbations or hospitalization for treatments, they are engrossed with the details and symptoms of the disease process and its life-threatening implications (clinical standard of health). When they are in remission or have a favorable treatment prognosis, they give more attention to concerns about work and family involvements (role-performance standard). All people with cancer are required to meet new challenges and develop new strategies for coping (adaptive standard); most patients, at some point in their odyssey, question the significance of their experience and its relevance in a cosmic scheme (eudaemonistic standard).

In summary, the challenge faced by professionals committed to improving the psychotherapeutic aspects of cancer care is to demonstrate effective approaches to help persons with cancer deal with the real and anticipated losses incurred in living with the disease. Universal conflict situations, the substantive base of time-limited psychotherapy, offer conceptual direction for exploring this very human concern. Instead of the question of the last two decades—"How can we support you while you are dying?"—now more and more we are asking "How can we help you to live as fully as possible under the conditions imposed by cancer and its treatments?" The emphasis in psychosocial oncology has shifted from preoccupation with dying to concern with living. In some ways, this changing focus on how to live and grow through loss signals new courage for all of us.

REFERENCES

BRONOWSKI, J. 1965. *Science and Human Values.* New York: Harper and Row.

MANN, J. 1973. *Time-Limited Psychotherapy.* Cambridge, MA: Harvard University Press.

MANN, J. AND R. GOLDMAN. 1982. *A Casebook in Time-Limited Therapy.* New York: McGraw-Hill..

RAWNSLEY, M. 1982. "Brief Psychotherapy for Persons with Recurrent Cancer: A Holistic Practice Model." *Advances in Nursing Science* 5(1):69–76.

SMITH, J. 1983. *The Idea of Health.* New York: Columbia University Press.

THOMAS, L. 1974. *The Lives of a Cell.* New York: Viking Press.

WINNICOTT, D. 1965. *Maturational Processes and the Facilitating Environment: Studies in the Theory of Emotional Development.* Madison, CT: International Universities Press.

23

When Your Dying Becomes My Dying: Aspects of Caregiver's Grief

Mary Dee McEvoy, RN, PhD

Let me begin by telling a story of an encounter I had with a patient. Mary S. was a 70-year-old female diagnosed with hypernephroma in June, 1984. In July, she had a right nephrectomy and in December, liver metastasis was discovered. She also developed a nodule above the operative site, which was diagnosed as adenocarcinoma. In April, 1985, she was admitted to a hospice unit, alert but disoriented as to time. Her pain was relieved by oral Dilaudid. Mary's husband said that she was aware of her diagnosis and was predominantly concerned about pain control.

Mary had worked as a file clerk all of her life, living with her husband, Roy, in a one-bedroom apartment in the Bronx. They had no children. She was of Italian descent and spoke Italian and English.

I began interacting with Mary about two weeks prior to her death. She was in a semicomatose state, talking for only brief periods. Roy visited daily for four to five hours. He really missed Mary and spoke of how difficult it was for him to return to the apartment each night.

Roy and I would sit together, one on each side of Mary. Sporadically, he would get up and move around, fidgeting with Mary's things, and then sit down and tell her how much he loved her. He talked with me about his father's and mother's deaths and some of the things that had happened to him.

He was originally from Sweden. He felt that he was pretty much of a stoic, and yet he would cry quite freely. He told me that I looked exactly like his mother and that he felt that he had his mother with him now to help him through this difficult time. I cried.

He talked about his life with Mary, how he was always sorry that they never had children. When Mary got angry with him, she would yell at him in Italian, calling him big and stupid. Then he would kiss her and tell her he loved her. She was totally bald, but Roy didn't mind—he kissed her on the head anyway.

Mary died on June 21, 1985. Roy cried and I cried. This was a death that I truly grieved.

Now, let us look more closely at this response to a patient's death. We will include an examination of personal responses to dying, a framework for the development of the caregiver, factors inhibiting the grieving process, and suggestions for dealing with grief.

PERSONAL RESPONSES TO DYING

Thomas Flynn (1986) has presented a framework for examining responses to dying. For Flynn, dying is a paradox: death is an abstraction, yet my death certainly is not; death is natural, but my death is anything but natural. This paradox can be examined by defining dying in terms of first, second, and third person.

Dying in the third person occurs when death is talked about in abstract terms, as when we teach about death. For most readers, the story of Mary S. would be death in the third person.

In contrast, death in the first person is my own death. This focuses on the uniqueness of the experience, in that we can never truly know death until we experience it personally.

Death in the second person involves identification with the dying person and is seen in relation to death of loved ones. It implies that someone is as dear to me as I am to myself. It becomes a shared experience; we cannot free the other from the experience, but we try to share it. Because relationships are what makes us human, a part of us is dying when we participate in dying in the second person.

In my opinion, when we experience death of a patient in third person terms, we may experience some detached sadness. However, when we experience death of a patient as death in the second person, we truly grieve that death. In the story, I really began to know Mary through Roy's eyes and to know what that relationship was like. When she died, I felt a lot of pain. That pain helped me to understand her death as death in the second person and to realize that it would take some work to get through it.

Worden (1982) states that there are four tasks to mourning:

(1) To accept the reality of the loss;
(2) To experience the pain of grief;
(3) To adjust to an environment without the deceased; and
(4) To withdraw emotional energy and invest it in another.

These same tasks must also be accomplished by the health care worker. The growth and development of the professional will affect his or her ability to mourn.

GROWTH AND DEVELOPMENT OF THE CAREGIVER

Harper (1977) has developed a schema that reflects stages of development of the professional who works with the terminally ill. Stage I is *intellectualization* and is characterized by knowledge and anxiety. The initial confrontation is very intellectual. There is a focus on professional knowledge, on factual as well as philosophical issues. Periods of brisk activity are incorporated into this stage as the caregiver focuses on understanding the environment, policies, and procedures. There is withdrawal from patients and families; the caregivers feel that death is unacceptable and therefore, while they may feel concerned about the patients, they are still uncomfortable.

Emotional survival is the thrust of Stage II, which is characterized by trauma, guilt, and frustration. As caregivers confront a patient's death, a confrontation with their own death occurs. Death is felt on an emotional level. Caregivers feels pity for the patient, leading to guilt and frustration as they compare their own health with the patient's illness. As the patient's death and possible suffering begins to be seen as unavoidable, hostility sets in.

Stage III, *depression,* is characterized by pain, mourning, and grief. This stage is crucial in terms of the growth of the caregiver. There is growing acceptance of the reality of death and an understanding that the feeling of frustration will not make it go away. In this stage, the caregiver either accepts the reality of death or goes on to another specialty.

Emotional arrival is Stage IV, characterized by moderation and accomodation. There is a sense of freedom from previous stages. Caregivers are free from identifying with the patient's symptoms and are no longer preoccupied with their own death. There are no guilt feelings and they are not incapacitated by depression. Although pain is still felt, they are free from the incapacitating effects of the pain. The caregivers are able to grieve and can recover.

Stage V, *deep compassion,* is characterized by self-realization and self-awareness. This stage is a culmination of all previous growth. Caregivers can relate compassionately to the dying patient with full acceptance of the impending death. Their work is enhanced by the dignity and self-respect they have for themselves, and this is transferred to the patient.

To superimpose the concepts of Flynn here, I would venture to say that, in Stage I, dying is seen in terms of the third person, with Stage III onward permitting dying in the second person.

David Popoff (1975), in an analysis of nurses' attitudes toward dying, relates several quotes. I note here two of them that reflect different developmental stages:

> My anger is usually misdirected. I get angry at the patient for being so demanding, at the family for not understanding, at the doctor for allowing him to suffer, and at my coworkers for being uncaring. I suspect the real object of my anger is my own inability to deal with these and other problems at times. (Respondent #9305)

This example reflects Stage II of development, while the following example is a Stage III or more:

> In caring for dying patients, the one predominant attitude I have developed is this: Life is too short; I must enjoy each day, get the most out of each moment, and live life to the fullest. I can now find happiness in many seemingly small things, where I couldn't before. I feel that my exposure to death and dying has made me realize the importance and joy of living. (Respondent #6900).

FACTORS INHIBITING GRIEVING

Although it is understood that professionals do grieve, and indeed, that grieving is viewed as a developmental characteristic, there are multiple factors that inhibit the grieving process. Consider the following:

(1) Social negation of the loss; the loss of a patient may not be viewed by coworkers as a reason to grieve.
(2) Social isolation; the opportunity for peer support may be minimal.
(3) Role of the strong one; when others are grieving, caregivers feel they must be strong.
(4) Feelings of ambivalence and guilt; there is a conflicting wish to cure as well as to see relief of suffering.
(5) Feeling of being overwhelmed by multiple losses. The concept of bereavement overload, usually referring to the multiple bereavements of the elderly, can also be applied to professionals.
(6) The reawakening of an old loss is always possible.

SUGGESTIONS FOR COPING

With the understanding of multiple grieving as part of the health professional's work, what are some strategies for dealing with this stress? Terese Rando (1984 pp. 440–443) suggests the following:

(1) Be aware of your feelings and be honest about them. Feelings are warning signs that physical and emotional limits have been met. Such feelings might be anger, disgust, exhaustion, and cynicism.

(2) Develop an awareness of your energy levels.

(3) Know your own feelings and attitudes toward dying.

(4) Identify stresses that are most troublesome.

(5) Be aware of how much you can reasonably accomplish with a given patient.

(8) Identify gaps in knowledge.

(9) Take care of physical needs, including relaxation.

(10) Develop decompression routines; this includes activities scheduled between work and home, such as exercise.

(11) Engage in life-affirming activities, such as play.

Pick Connor (1986) suggests the use of a journal in writing down personal thoughts, fears, and concerns that might be involved in grief work.

*   *   *

Let us return now to the story. For me this was definitely a case of dying in the second person. I felt very strongly for Mary and Roy and felt that a part of me had definitely changed because of them. I think that I may have been moving through Stage III to Stage IV; although I didn't have guilt feelings, I was somewhat incapacitated. For a while I didn't even realize that I was mourning. This was related to social isolation (I didn't use the peer support available) and assuming the role of the strong one (I was viewed as an expert and perceived as strong). The technique I used to realize my grief work was the use of a journal.

REFERENCES

CONNOR, P. 1986. "Guided Journal Work as an Aid to Resolving Grief." Paper presented at the Eighth Annual Conference of the Forum for Death Education and Counseling, April.

FLYNN, T. 1986. "Dying as Doing: Some Philosophical Reflections on Death and Authenticity." Paper presented at the Eighth Annual Conference of the Forum for Death Education and Counseling, April.

HARPER, B. 1977. "Schematic Growth and Development Scale in Coping with Professional Anxieties in Terminal Illness." In *The Coping Mechanisms of the Health Professional.* Greenville, SC: Southeastern University Press.

POPOFF, D. 1975. "What Are Your Feelings About Death and Dying?" *Nursing* 5(8):15–24

RANDO, T. 1984. *Grief, Dying and Death: Clinical Interventions for Caregivers.* Champaign, IL: Research Press Co.

WORDEN, J. 1982. *Grief Counseling and Grief Therapy.* New York: Springer.

24

A Comparison of the Terminally Ill Cancer Patient's Perception of Needs vs. the Perceptions of the Family and the Nurse

Matthew Bellanich, MS, RN

> You see, you start from a completely false position. No sooner does
> a patient come to you than you begin to do all his thinking for him.
> After that, the thinking's done by your standing orders, your five-
> minute conferences, your program, your plan and the honor of your
> medical department. And once again I become a grain of sand, just
> as I was in the camp. Once again nothing depends on me.
> —*Cancer Ward* (Alexander Solzhenitsyn 1969)

This chapter identifies how the patient, family, and nurse view the needs of
the hospitalized, terminally ill cancer patient. It looks at the perceptions dying
patients have of their nursing needs. The perceptions of the family and nurse
are also identified. Congruent patterns of perception and communication
between these three groups are discussed.

The following assumptions are made:

1. Social supports influence an individual's perception (Caplan 1964).
2. Communication is a dimension of perception.
3. Congruence between reported perceptions of the patient's needs by the
   patient, family, and nurse indicates clear communication between these
   groups.
4. The needs of the terminally ill in the hospital are subject to the
   organizational and social needs of the institution (Blauner 1966;
   Mauksch 1975; Benoliel 1976; Kastenbaum 1976).

211

5. Persons who are dying have special needs (Quint 1967; Parsons 1977).

The following hypotheses are made:

1. Patients in the hospital, dying of cancer, will perceive their needs differently than nurses perceive their needs.
2. Patients in the hospital, dying of cancer, will perceive their needs differently than families perceive their needs.
3. Nurses' and families' perceptions of hospitalized, terminally ill cancer patient's needs will be more similar to each other than to the patients' perceptions.

In operationally defining the terms of this analysis, *patient's needs* are measured by an adaptation of the Shorupka Q-Sort (Skorupka and Bohnet 1982), with 18 additional items designed by the investigator. The *patient* is a person with a diagnosis of cancer of more than four months duration, and with confirmation of metastatic disease (Parsons 1977). The *family* member is a blood relative, spouse, or significant other. The *nurse* is a registered nurse who had provided care for the patient on at least two occasions. The *hospital* setting is a large, acute, care, teaching institution.

This chapter seeks to examine the attitudes toward, and understanding of, nursing care for the terminal cancer patient. How has the level of communication between the patient, family, and nurse been affected by the isolating experience of dying? Where do perceptions agree, and where do they differ?

Theoretical Framework: Rosel's conceptual framework on the social aspects of dying (1979) provides the theoretical framework. Three aspects of dying are addressed: effective coping, control over death, and socialization of the dying.

The dying must deal with both physical losses and separation losses. Physical comfort measures and open communications are means of helping the dying cope effectively, setting up patterns and expectations that assist in defining a role for the dying. The dying seek to obtain some control over death, a goal with which institutions are frequently incompatable. The dying cannot be socialized into a dying role, nor are there roles to support those who provide for their care.

Review of the Literature: Weisman and Hackett (1961) wrote how the attitudes of isolation, silence, deception, and denial of the terminal nature of an illness frequently resulted in suffering, loneliness, withdrawal, and a sense of emotional abandonment for the patient. Open communication was identified as an essential element in altering the patient's attitude toward death so that motivation and ego function can be maintained until death prevails. Like Weisman and Hackett, Glaser and Strauss (1965) saw that open, shared awareness that acknowledges the patient is dying lessens withdrawal and isolation. Communication patterns that foster isolation lead to the loss of direct communications with the patient, and the patient is treated as if he were already dead (Kastenbaum 1965). Parsons' (1977) study on the preceptions of dying patients' needs demonstrated that such patients could still enjoy life, given a supportive atmosphere. However, studies by Glaser and Strauss (1964), Quint (1967), Krant and Payne (1969), Stoller (1981), and Gow (1982) support the findings that professional caregivers, in an attempt to distance themselves emotionally from the dying, can thereby increase the dying person's feeling of isolation. Furthermore, studies by Jennings and Muhlenkamp (1981) and Lauer, Murray, and Powers (1982) demonstrate a misperception by nurses of the affective, as well as cognitive, needs of the dying.

Setting and Sample: This study was conducted at Boston University Medical Center, a large, inner-city teaching institution. The sample population consisted of patients on oncology units. All had metastatic disease of more than six months duration, with a mean duration of 24 months. Patients were selected by chronological admission. All but five patients had been hospitalized longer than two days, with the average hospitalization being 15.4 days. A post-study survey revealed that 13 patients (57 percent) had died within three months of the completion of the data collection.

Spouses and daughters represented 74 percent of family participants. Most families were Irish, and three-fourths were Catholic.

Three-quarters of the registered nurses participating (n-19) were under 30 years old. Only three nurses did not have their B.S.N., and only two had less than one year experience caring for terminal patients. Thirty seven percent had two to three years experience. Sixty-five percent of the nurses had a professional relationship with the patient of greater than six months duration.

METHODOLOGY

Instrument: This cross sectional study utilized a Q-sort methodology. Forty-one items from the Skorupka Q-Sort were adapted for this study. Skorupka's tool was developed to evaluate the needs of oncology nurses in catagories of patients' physical and psychosocial needs, and nurses' psychosocial needs. Only items dealing with patients' needs were included in this study. These items were reworded to reflect a patient's preception. Each statement was reconstructed so as to retain the nursing behavior contained in the Skorupka Q-Sort. Eighteen additional items, based on a review of the literature, were added to ensure statistical stability with the Q-sort methodology. These items also reflected both physical and psychosocial needs of the dying patient.

Validity: The content validity of the Skorupka Q-Sort had previously been determined by six nursing experts in the content area.

Content validity for the items constructed by the investigator was determined by five nursing educators with masters and doctoral preparation, and three hospice nurses. There was 100 percent agreement on all items.

Procedure: These 59 nursing behaviors were typed on individual cards. Each participant was asked to choose the 15 most and least helpful items for that particular patient. While most unstructured Q-sorts are sorted on a continuum, indicating degrees of desirability, only the extreme ends of the continuum were used in this study. By constructing an artificial dichotomy of least, most, and neutral behaviors, the congruence of perception could still be tested. This adaption was less complex and more suitable for very ill patients.

Family members and nurses were asked to complete the Q-sort. In four cases, nurses completed the Q-sort on two different patients.

Limitations: As a nonrandom sample, generalizations beyond this sample cannot be made. A religious and cultural skew further restrict any generalizations beyond the sample.

FINDINGS

Using Spearman's Rank Order Coefficient, significant correlations were demonstrated between the patient-family groups (p .01). Correlation was highly significant in the area of most desirable nursing actions. A rho value of .679 (p .001) was obtained. A value of .574 (p .01) was seen for the patient–family groups in the area of least helpful behaviors.

Hypothesis 1 was supported by these findings, although Hypothesis 2 was not. Patients saw their needs differently than did nurses, but there was a significant level of agreement with these families. Nurses and family members did not share similar perceptions; therefore, Hypothesis 3 was not supported.

In the analysis of the descriptive data, the 59 behaviors were catagorized into McGrory's eight areas of need for the dying (1979). They are: improving communication, facilitating grief work, relieving pain, providing physical care, maintaining a positive body image, providing an opportunity for life review, ensuring spiritual comfort, and managing the environment.

Communication Needs: All three groups felt that responding to a patient's question honestly was important. However, it is interesting to note that, while 61 percent of the patients felt this way, 26 percent of the patients did not see this as important. All groups tended to see a need to keep the patient informed, but again, 30 percent of the patients did not value being informed. On the other hand, 44 percent of the family members questioned did not feel that the nurse should encourage the patient to ask questions.

All the groups saw a need to encourage hope. The patient and family groups even supported offering false hope. Encouraging hope, however, was felt to be least helpful to their patients by 22 percent of the nurses.

Nurses tended to see themselves as sources of support for the family. Patients and family, though, disagreed.

All groups supported behaviors that favored emotional support of the patient. Nurses, in an overwhelming majority (83 percent), identified the expression of feelings by the patient as helpful. However, 22 percent of nurses did not feel that staying with patients when they were having difficulty was helpful.

Only one patient felt the distraction of talking about things other than their disease was very helpful to them. In contrast, 48 percent of nurses and 35 percent of families placed high value on such distraction.

Grief Work: When the behaviors dealing with grief were addressed in general terms, such as helping the patient to cope with anxiety from a progressive disease or from the disappointment of setbacks, all groups tended to value the support of the nurse. However, specific behaviors such as crying, grieving, and talking about death and dying were not viewed as helpful by the patient–family groups. Only 17 percent of the nurses felt that allowing the patient to cry helped. Twenty-two percent felt crying was undesirable. Only 22 percent of nurses felt it was important to recognize when the patient wanted to talk about dying and death. Almost as many nurses (17 percent) identified this as least important. All groups saw little need to help the patient cope with physical losses.

Pain Control: Almost half the patients (44 percent) felt they needed support to accept pain medication as often as necessary, yet 26 percent of the nurses did not see this as helping, and only 13 percent agreed with this patient perception. While all groups were in favor of keeping the patient comfortable, family members were most concerned (70 percent), and nurses were least concerned (30 percent). Half the patients saw pain control as their priority.

Physical Care: Patients and families tended to place a strong emphasis on the nurse providing physical, rehabilitative, and emergency care for the patient. One-third of the nurses felt that maxamizing physical function, rehabilitation, assisting with activities of daily living, and helping the patient to stay active and out of bed were least helpful to the patient. While appearing to favor bed rest for these patients, 61 percent of the nurses saw little need to prevent complications of long-term bed rest.

Self-Esteem: Most nurses (52–70 percent) felt that patients should adapt to their situation at their own pace, be included in planning their care, have their decisions and choices supported, and have their concerns listened to. While half of the patients and families felt it was important to have the patient's concerns listened to, they were much less supportive of these other actions. All groups felt there was little need to help the patient feel useful to others.

Life Review: All three groups felt there was little need to help the patients conclude relationships and activities in their lives. Most patients and family members also felt that recalling life events was unhelpful. Though more than one-third of the nurses agreed with this perception, another third felt a life review was important.

Spiritual Needs: All groups strongly agreed that the patient's spiritual life was not an area for nursing intervention. Behaviors related to the patient's spiritual life produced some of the strongest and most uniform responses of this study.

Environmental Needs: Few nurses felt that actions that promoted a clean, neat, pleasant environment were helpful to the patient. Most nurses (39–65 percent) felt this to be the least helpful. Patients and family tended to be more evenly split as to how important this was to them.

CONCLUSION

The avoidance by the nurses of both intimate behaviors and physical actions, as well as their inability to offer hope, suggests that they may feel unsupported in their task of caring for the dying patient. There is a sense of emotional withdrawal and inability to deal with issues of loss on the part of the nurses.

Nurses need to be better prepared to help patients and families deal with loss. This can occur only if nurses are attuned to their own feelings of loss and hope.

The process must begin with education. Dying—both the personal experience and the biological process—must be better understood through the sharing of attitudes, feelings, and knowledge. We must listen to our patients, for what we need to learn, patients may already know.

The process must continue with support. Institutions must recognize their mission of caring, not just curing. They must reevaluate the priorities they place on supporting the dying and on supporting those who are called upon to carry out that mission of support.

REFERENCES

BENOLIEL, J. Q. 1976. "Overview: Care, Cure, and the Challenge of Choice." In A.M. Earle, N.T. Aogodizzo, and A.H. Kutscher, eds, *The Nurse Caregiver for the Terminal Patient and His Family.* New York: Columbia University Press.

BLAUNER, R. 1966. "Death and Social Structure." *Psychiatry* 29(1):378–394.

CAPLAN, G. 1964. *Principles of Preventive Psychiatry.* New York: Basic Books, Inc.

GLASER, B., AND A. STRAUSS. 1964. "The Social Loss of Dying Patients." *American Journal of Nursing* 64(6):119–121.

GLASER, B., AND A. STRAUSS. 1965. *Awareness of Dying.* Chicago: Adline.

GOW, K. M. 1982. *How Nurses' Emotions Affect Patient Care: Self Studies by Nurses.* New York: Springer Publishing Co.

JENNINGS, B. M. AND A. F. MUHLENKAMP. 1981. "Systematic Misperception: Oncology Patients' Self-Reported Affective States and their Caregivers' Perceptions." *Cancer Nursing* 4(6):485–489.

KASTENBAUM, R. 1969. "Psychological Death." In L. Pearsons, ed. *Death and Dying.* Cleveland: The Press of Case Western Reserve University.

KASTENBAUM, R. 1976. "Toward Standards of Care for the Terminally Ill, Part III: A Few Guiding Principles." *Omega* 7(3):191–193.

KRANT, M. J., AND E. C. PAYNE., 1969. "Interviewing Cancer Patients." *Journal of the American Medical Association* 210(7):1239–1242.

LAUER, P., S. MURPHY, AND M. POWERS, 1982. "Learning Needs of Cancer Patients: A Comparison of Nurse and Patient Perceptions." *Nursing Research* 31(10):11–16.

MAUKSCH, H. O. 1975. "The Organizational Context of Dying." In E. KublerRoss, ed. *Death, the Final Stage of Growth.* Englewood Cliffs, N.J.: Prentice-Hall.

MCGRORY, A. 1978. *A Well Model Approach to Care of the Dying Patient.* New York: McGraw-Hill.

PARSONS, J. 1977. "A Descriptive Study of Intermediate State Terminally Ill Cancer Patients at Home." *Nursing Digest* 5(2):1–26.

QUINT, J. C. 1967. *The Nurse and the Dying Patient.* New York: Macmillan.

ROSEL, N. 1979. "Toward a Social Theory of Dying." *Omega* 9(1):49–55.

SKORUPKA, P., AND N. BOHNET. 1982. "Primary Caregivers' Perceptions of Nursing Behaviors that Best Meet Their Needs in a Home Care Hospice Setting." *Cancer Nursing* 5(5):371–374.

SOLZHENITSYN, A. 1969. *Cancer Ward.* New York: Grosset and Dunlap.

STOLLER, E. 1981. "The Impact of Death Related Fears on Attitudes of Nurses in a Hospital Work Setting." *Omega* 11(1):85–96.

WEISMAN, A., AND T. HACKETT. 1961. "Predilection to Death." *Psychosomatic Medicine* 23(3):232–256.

25

Humor as a Teaching Strategy for Caregivers

Christine A. Rovinski, RN, MSN

Student nurses are normally reticent when introduced to new clinical rotations whose focus is on mental health. During orientation to psychosocial cancer care, particularly the terminal aspect, this reticence is often amplified. Preconceived ideas and life experiences with the disease typically overwhelm even the most proficient students. They are immobilized by their own psychological pain. Their anxieties about working with the oncology population on a feelings level are manifested by a concentration on physical tasks rather than on the patients.

One strategy for dealing with this response is humor, which alters one's perspective by challenging the integrity of an accepted reality. For example, most people are not inclined toward appreciation of "dead baby jokes." Therefore, such a joke shared during clinical conference is guaranteed to spark an active discussion about idiosyncratic relationships with death-themed topics.

The horrible nature of the joke, the dramatic violation of the norm, can establish a bond between the students and the instructor. Through the instructor's irreverent role-modeling, the students are encouraged to entertain new and unstructured thoughts about the joke's content.

There is an intense expression of feelings as inhibitions relax. Excitement peaks as students explore the absurd, unhampered by any restrictions in the cognitive process. The students test and compare their own value systems under the nonthreatening pretext of examining the reactions of others to the joke. The frivolity ebbs as they begin to understand that the selection of one's reality is a subjective, and sometimes arbitrary, process. With this, their anxieties diminish to a level over which they can exert an effective control.

The nursing student's ability to understand his or her personal pattern of adaptation is an important adjunct to the satisfactory performance of psychosocial patient care. As self-awareness increases, so does perception of the available options for purposeful interaction with the cancer patient. The student recognizes that the basic principles of therapeutic communication are consistent, regardless of the clinical setting. Behaviors become aligned with constructive reasoning. No longer emotionally pained, the student becomes increasingly client-centered and demonstrates strengthened competency in the techniques of psychosocial cancer nursing.

The comic approach in education should tailor the humor to desired outcome behaviors, which are defined prior to the clinical rotation. Jokes, cartoons, and anecdotes must receive as much attention to detail as the more conventional content. They must fit into the learning situation and not seem forced. Their use as formal content material must take into account the preferences of other people, so that the humor is not derogatory.

An important goal is the student's socialization within the oncology setting. When attuned to the adaptive functions of comedy, the instructor has access to one of the student's most accurate portrayals of his or her psychosocial connectedness.

Humor presupposes a common language. In cancer care, gallows humor predominates. Identification of what makes students laugh in that genre, as well as what doesn't, exposes their vulnerabilities.

What is the student's response to the staff nurses who accept the elderly woman's invitation to pat her chemo-induced baldness for luck before they select their lottery numbers? Does it repel the student, or is it seen as an expression of the patient's need for physical contact and reassurance that she retains a place in everyday activities? Can the student appreciate that the confrontation with a frustrating reality has been couched to encourage interaction, and that there is a reaffirmation of normalcy within the bizarre?

The student's responses are indicative of his or her baseline frame of reference. Does the student laugh when the instructor relates the experience of finding a corpse frozen in a getting-out-of-bed position? What is the student's reaction to hearing that "Doctor, please reorder" tape was used to keep the shroud closed and that the body was rocked like a cradle to make sure it was securely fastened? Is the student shocked at the behaviors? How well does he or she solve the dilemma of being stuck at midnight with a corpse that won't fit into the morgue refrigerator and a morgue attendant who won't accept the body until it does? What is the student's reaction to the instructor's willingness to disclose less-than-exemplary nursing practice?

The instructor should also be alert to student-initiated humor. Is it compatible with the humor that is generally produced and sanctioned on the unit? One student shared a Charles Addams-type greeting card with staff members who regarded their designation as oncology nurses as something akin to a mission from God. Rather than the cameraderie she expected, the student was subjected to a day of mutterings about her insensitivity. Alternately, a hospice staff reacted gleefully after another student targeted their frustration with the local funeral parlors. She suggested that the hospice use shrouds imprinted ''From our house to yours.'' Knowing each student's fluency with the language of emotional survival in an oncology setting helps the instructor determine individual prescriptions for student development.

One nursing school has a large number of students from the Caribbean. Many of these students fear death, believe in voodoo, and fully expect the dead to rise. As a result, their initial exposure to imminent death and postmortem care is unusually stressful. Humorous accounts of the instructor's experiences with postmortem care have proved beneficial in identifying cultural fears, dispelling myths, and supporting student ability to cope appropriately when in close physical proximity to a dying person or a corpse.

In a social situation, the listener judges the success of the humor. In a academic setting, the instructor evaluates its effectiveness. The successful application of humor was measured with the West Indian students by the increase in the number of student-initiated requests to sit with dying clients, by a decrease in the number of students who bolted from a patient's room the first time a corpse moaned or moved spontaneously, by the reduction in the histrionics that previously characterized clinical assignments in the oncology setting, and by the decreased use of monté (silver rings, chains, and medals that have previously been treated by the *ougan* or witch doctor to ward off evil spirits and zombies).

Nursing students in the cancer care setting need to acquire psychosocial skills that are useful for the immediate present and for the future. They need to learn how to cope constructively with frustration, how to critically self-analyze without destroying self-confidence, and how not to run away from empathic contact.

The comic approach meets these needs. It helps students deal with the emotional stress of the cancer care environment by providing an acceptable outlet for thoughts and feelings that may not be congruent with the oncology setting. Humor promotes creativity and an exhilarating sense of discovery that makes learning desirable. The nursing instructor who uses humor has many opportunities to direct the student's cognitive reorganization, motivate the process of self-awareness, purposefully guide confrontations with reality, and measure the student's acclimation to the cancer care environment.

SUGGESTED READING

BUTTERFIELD, S. 1985. "Professional Nursing Education: What Is Its Purpose?" *Journal of Nursing Education* 24(3): 99–103.

CARPENITO, L.J. AND T.A. DUESPOHL. 1981. *A Guide for Effective Clinical Instruction.* Rockville, Maryland: Aspen Systems Corporation.

COHEN, S.J. 1985. "Laughter and High Level Wellness." *Health Values* 9(4): 32.

HARKINS-MCNARY, L.H. 1979. "The Use of Humor in Group Therapy." *Perspectives in Psychiatric Care* 17(5): 228–231.

HENDERSON, V. 1961. *The Nature of Nursing: A Definition and Its Implications for Practice, Research and Education.* New York: The Macmillan Company.

HERTH, K.A 1984. "Laughter: A Nursing Rx" *American Journal of Nursing* 84(8): 991–992.

JACOBSEN, B.S. 1983. "A Statistical Tale of Significance." *Nursing Research* 32(6): 376–377.

JOURARD, S.M. 1971. *The Transparent Self.* New York: Van Nostrand Reinhold Company.

OSTERLAND, H. 1983. "Humor: A Serious Approach to Nursing Care." *Nursing* 13(12): 46–47.

ROBINSON, V. 1978. "Humor." In C. Carlson and B. Blackwell, eds. *Behavioral Concepts and Nursing Interventions.* New York: J. B. Lippincott Company.

SCHWEER, J.E AND K.M. GEBBIE. 1976. *Creative Teaching in Clinical Nursing.* St. Louis: The C.V. Mosby Company.

TOPPER, V.A. 1985. "Improving Your Laugh Life." *Nursing Life* 5(2): 58–61.

WARNER, S.L. 1984. "Humor and Self-Disclosure Within the Milieu." *Journal of Psychosocial Nursing* 22(4):17–21.

26

The Search for an Institutional Approach to Thanatology in a Cancer Center

Yall Silverberg, PhD, Frank Adams, Donna R. Copeland, Wayne L. Dorris, Helmuth Goepfert, Joel K. Levi, John F. Stelling, Kathleen R. Stevens, and Louise Villejos

In an attempt to develop an institutional approach to thanatology for the University of Texas System Cancer Center, M.D. Anderson Hospital and Tumor Institute, we conducted a survey of all U.S. Comprehensive Cancer Centers in order to find out the nature and extent of their activities in this area. This chapter relates the results of that survey. It constitutes a step in the background search for a unified approach to the subject at the University of Texas Cancer Center (UTCC), M.D. Anderson Hospital and Tumor Institute. Present activities at M.D. Anderson Hospital are related and discussed against this background. Suggestions for future activities and research follow.

A MEDLINE search of the HEALTH database covering the period 1975–1985 for the term "Thanatology" identified 58 citations. *A Comprehensive Bibliography of the Thanatology Literature*, (Kutscher et al. 1975) lists 4844 references in 424 categories. Simpson's *Dying, Death, and Grief: A Bibliography and Source Book of Thanatology and Terminal Care*, published in 1979, carefully describes 708 publications and rates them in five levels from "not recommended, not suitable for use at all" to "strongly recommended, buy and read." It appears that the thanatology literature is voluminous. It includes many categories and, according to Simpson (1979) varies widely in quality and usefulness. Situations involving death and dying are ever present in cancer centers. However, an example of a unified institutional approach to the subject was not found in this literature search.

MATERIALS AND METHODS

A thanatology-related activities questionnaire, designed to obtain information about present approaches to thanatology in all U.S. Comprehensive Cancer Centers, was developed by representatives of interested departments at M.D. Anderson Hospital. The questionnaire was pretested in the departments of Chaplaincy, Neuropsychiatry, Nursing, Patient Education and Social Work. These departments were asked to submit detailed descriptions of past and current thanatology-related activities. They were also requested to project their plans for future activities in this area. The questionnaire included six questions directed at finding out whether thanatology was presented as a part of the formal training/educational programs, and if research was conducted on reactions to death, loss and grief, and recovery from bereavement.

Since comprehensive cancer centers include multidisciplinary professional staff, the questionnaire was administered to a number of involved subpopulations of professionals in order to gauge the extent of their involvement in thanatology-related activities. Frequencies and proportions of activities were calculated for each subpopulation at M.D. Anderson and, based on the data received, for the responding cancer centers.

Following the survey at M.D. Anderson Hospital during February–April, 1986, the questionnaire was mailed to the directors of all 21 U.S. Comprehensive Cancer Centers. However, detailed descriptions of their future plans were not requested. The data collected were analyzed for all cancer centers as a group and then, separately, for M.D. Anderson Hospital.

RESULTS

U.S. Comprehensive Cancer Centers: The 16 of 21 U.S. Comprehensive Cancer Centers responding to the survey accounted for a 76.2 percent response rate. Table 1 enumerates the responding centers reporting inclusion of thanatology topics in their training/education. Nurses' training/education addressed the topic in 11 (68.8 percent) of the responding cancer centers. Nine 56.8 percent centers) included the topic in the training of their social workers, and eight (50 percent) incorporated it in the educational programs for the clergy and medical students. Training/education programs of residents and fellows included thanatology-related topics in seven (43.8 percent) of the responding centers. For relatives of patients it was included in six (37.5 percent) of the responding centers, and in programs for staff physicians in five (31.3 percent) centers. LVN's received thanatology euducation/training in four (25 percent) of the responding centers.

Table 1

U.S. Comprehensive Cancer Centers Including Thanatology Related Topics As Part Of Their Training/Educational Programs, 1985-86

Populations	Comprehensive Cancer Centers	Total No.	Percent
Medical students	a,b, d, f,g j, m,n	8	50.0
Residents	b, d, f,g j, m,n	7	43.8
Fellows	b, d, f,g j, m,n	7	43.8
Staff physicians	b, d, f,g j	5	31.3
Nurses	a,b,c,d, f,g i,j,k, m,n	11	68.8
LVN's	d, f,g m	4	25.0
Social workers	b,c,d, f,g,h,i,j m	9	56.3
Clergy	c,d, f,g,h, j,k, m	8	50.0
Patients' relatives	b, f,g j,k, m	6	37.5
Other (specify)	d, f,g i	4	25.0

a.	Columbia	g.	Mayo
b.	Dana-Farber	h.	Memorial-Sloan Kettering
c.	Duke	i.	Michigan
d.	Fox Chase	j.	Papanicolaou
e.	Fred Hutchinson	k.	Roswell Park Memorial
f.	M. D. Anderson		

l.	Ohio State U.
m.	U. of Alabama
n.	USC
o.	Univ. Wisconsin
p.	Yale

Thanatology related topics, in addition to being included by cancer centers in formal training/education programs for their subpopulations, are often addressed in lectures, symposia, grand rounds, and patient education. Table 2 identifies the centers reporting these activities for their various subpopulations. Fourteen (87.5 percent) indicated offering some of these activities to nurses, ten (62.5 percent) to social workers, and nine (56.3 percent) to the clergy. Medical students, fellows, and staff physicians encountered these activities in eight (50 percent) centers, while seven institutions (43.8 percent) offered them to residents and six (25 percent) to patients' relatives. Two centers (12.5 percent) extended these activities to other populations.

Table 3 lists the cancer centers in which research on reactions to death and dying has been conducted. Of the 16 responding centers, one (6.3 percent) reported having conducted such research with the clergy, one (6.3 percent) with patients and one (6.3 percent) with other populations.

Research on the psychological aspects of dying (Table 4) was reported with

Table 2

U.S. Comprehensive Cancer Centers Offering
Thanatology-Related Lectures/Symposia/Grand Rounds/
Patient Education to Their Subpopulations, 1985-86

Populations	Comprehensive Cancer Centers	Total No.	Percent
Medical students	a, d, f,g j,k,l,m	8	50.0
Residents	a, d, f,g j,k,l	7	43.8
Fellows	a, d, f,g j,k,l o	8	50.0
Staff physicians	a, c,d, f,g j, n,o	8	50.0
Nurses	a,b,c,d,e,f,g j,k,l,m,n,o,p	14	87.5
LVN's	a, c,d, f,g m	6	37.5
Social workers	a,b,c,d,e,f,g j, l,m	10	62.5
Clergy	a, c,d, f,g j,k, m, o,	9	56.3
Patients	a, c, f,g j n	6	37.5
Patients' relatives	a, c, f, n	4	25.0
Other (specify)	f,g	2	12.5

a.	Columbia	g.	Mayo
b.	Dana-Farber	h.	Memorial-Sloan Kettering
c.	Duke	i.	Michigan
d.	Fox Chase	j.	Papanicolaou
e.	Fred Hutchinson	k.	Roswell Park Memorial
f.	M. D. Anderson		

l. Ohio State U.
m. U. of Alabama
n. USC
o. Univ. Wisconsin
p. Yale

research was carried out with fellows, nurses, social workers, and the clergy, each in one (6.3 percent) separate center.

Table 5 shows where research on loss and grief took place. Three (18.8 percent) centers carried out such research with patients' relatives, one (6.3 percent) with the clergy, one (6.3 percent) with patients, and one (6.3 percent) with another population.

Cancer centers where research on recovery from bereavement took place are listed in Table 6. This research was done with nurses in three (18.8 percent) centers, with patients' relatives in two (12.5 percent) canters, and with social workers and clergy each in one (6.3 percent) separate center.

The University of Texas Cancer Center, M.D. Anderson Hospital and Tumor Institute: Table 7 lists the departments at M.D. Anderson Hospital offering thanatology-related topics as part of their training/education programs. Six departments indicated involvement in thanatology training/education programs with various subpopulations in the institution. The departments were:

Table 3

U.S. Comprehensive Cancer Centers Where Research of Reactions to Death and Dying Took Place with Various Populations During 1981-1985

Populations	Comprehensive Cancer Centers	Total No.	Percent
Medical students			
Residents			
Fellows			
Staff physicians			
Nurses			
LVN's			
Social workers			
Clergy	k,	1	6.3
Patients	h,	1	6.3
Patients' relatives			
Other (specify)	k,	1	6.3

a.	Columbia	g.	Mayo	l.	Ohio State U.
b.	Dana-Farber	h.	Memorial-Sloan Kettering	m.	U. of Alabama
c.	Duke	i.	Michigan	n.	USC
d.	Fox Chase	j.	Papanicolaou	o.	Univ. Wisconsin
e.	Fred Hutchinson	k.	Roswell Park Memorial	p.	Yale
f.	M. D. Anderson				

Chaplaincy, Nursing, Patient Education, Pediatrics, and Social Work. The Department of Nursing, which includes thanatology as a formal part of its training/education, is addressed by representatives of four (66.7 percent) other departments. Patients' relatives are addressed by three (50 percent) departments and LVN's by two (33.3 percent). Residents, fellows, social-work staff and three other subpopulations are instructed about thanatology by one (16.7 percent) department. It appears that the Chaplaincy is involved in thanatology instruction of seven (58.3 percent) subpopulations in the institution, Patient Education and Social Work each in the instruction of three (25 percent) subpopulations, Nursing in two (16.7 percent), and Pediatrics in one (8.3 percent).

As Table 8 demonstrates, the department of Pediatrics was most active in offering thanatology-related activities tailored to fit particular needs. Lectures about thanatology were offered by Pediatrics to nine of 13 (69.2 percent) subpopulations in the hospital. The department of Patient Education provided

Table 4

**U.S. Comprehensive Cancer Centers where Research of
the Psychological Aspects of Dying with Various
Subpopulations was carried out sometime
between 1981-1985**

Populations	Comprehensive Cancer Centers				Total No.	Percent
Medical students						
Residents						
Fellows	b,				1	6.3
Staff physicians						
Nurses		h,			1	6.3
LVN's						
Social workers		h,			1	6.3
Clergy			k,		1	6.3
Patients	b,	g,	j,	p,	4	25.0
Patients' relatives	b,	g,			2	12.5
Other (specify)						

a.	Columbia	g.	Mayo	l.	Ohio State U.
b.	Dana-Farber	h.	Memorial-Sloan Kettering	m.	U. of Alabama
c.	Duke	i.	Michigan	n.	USC
d.	Fox Chase	j.	Papanicolaou	o.	Univ. Wisconsin
e.	Fred Hutchinson	k.	Roswell Park Memorial	p.	Yale
f.	M. D. Anderson				

lectures to three (21.4 percent) subpopulations, and Nursing and Social Work each to one (7.7 percent) subpopulation. Symposia were organized by the Chaplaincy for three (23.1 percent) subpopulations in the hospital. The departments of Patient Education and the Chaplaincy offered thanatology-related patient education. The department of Patient Education extended these activities to four (30.8 percent) subpopulations and the Chaplaincy to one (7.7 percent).

Thanatology-related staffing conferences were conducted only by the department of Pediatrics. The conferences included representatives of 10 (71.4 percent) hospital subpopulations. Also unique to the Pediatrics department was an activity called Process Group Following Death, which was offered to representatives of 10 (71.4 percent) subpopulations in the hospital.

Read from a different direction, Table 8 also shows which departments offered what type of thanatology instruction to other subpopulation at the cancer

Table 5

U.S. Comprehensive Cancer Centers Where Research of Loss and Grief Took Place with Various Subpopulations Between 1981-1985

Populations	Comprehensive Cancer Centers	Total No.	Percent
Medical students			
Residents			
Fellows			
Staff physicians			
Nurses			
LVN's			
Social workers			
Clergy	k,	1	6.3
Patients	f,		6.3
Patients' relatives	f, h, m,	3	18.8
Other (specify)	k,	1	6.3

a.	Columbia	g.	Mayo	l.	Ohio State U.
b.	Dana-Farber	h.	Memorial-Sloan Kettering	m.	U. of Alabama
c.	Duke	i.	Michigan	n.	USC
d.	Fox Chase	j.	Papanicolaou	o.	Univ. Wisconsin
e.	Fred Hutchinson	k.	Roswell Park Memorial	p.	Yale
f.	M. D. Anderson				

center. It appears that the Nursing department received instruction from four of six (66.7 percent) departments involved in thanatology-related activities. Social workers and fellows-in-training were addressed by three of six (50 percent) departments; medical students, residents and the clergy by two of six (33.3 percent) departments; and staff physicians, patients' relatives, psychologists, child life workers, and translators each by one of six (16.7 percent) departments. The department of Pediatrics is the most active in offering thanatology instruction. It is followed by Patient Education and the Chaplaincy.

Preliminary plans for research of thanatology-related issues were reported only by the Chaplaincy. This research is to include patients and their relatives.

DISCUSSION

Response rate of all U.S. Comprehensive Cancer Centers was slightly above 76 percent. Responses were not received from five, or 23.8 percent, of the institutions in spite of repeated follow-up. Reasons for the lack of response remain obscure.

Table 6

U.S. Comprehensive Cancer Centers Where Research of Recovery from Bereavement Took Place with Various Subpopulations Between 1981-1985

Populations	Comprehensive Cancer Centers		Total No.	Percent
Medical students				
Residents				
Fellows				
Staff physicians				
Nurses	c,	m,n,	3	18.8
LVN's				
Social workers	h,		1	6.3
Clergy	k,		1	6.3
Patients				
Patients' relatives	h,	m,	2	12.5
Other (specify)				

a.	Columbia	g.	Mayo	l.	Ohio State U.
b.	Dana-Farber	h.	Memorial-Sloan Kettering	m.	U. of Alabama
c.	Duke	i.	Michigan	n.	USC
d.	Fox Chase	j.	Papanicolaou	o.	Univ. Wisconsin
e.	Fred Hutchinson	k.	Roswell Park Memorial	p.	Yale
f.	M. D. Anderson				

Training and Education: Thanatology is an integral part of training/educational programs for nurses in a large proportion of U.S. Cancer Centers. Fewer institutions, but still higher than 50 percent, include thanatology-related topics in the training/education of social workers. A surprisingly small proportion, 50 percent, include it in the training of the clergy and medical students. An even smaller proportion incorporate the topic in training of residents and fellows, and a mere 31 percent offer it to staff physicians. One may conclude therefore that thanatology training/education in U.S. Cancer Centers is directed mainly to nurses and social workers and least to LVN's and staff physicians.

This trend is consistent enough to suggest that, among caregivers in a cancer center, nurses and social workers receive the most extensive education and training about thanatology. Physicians and medical trainees are far less involved. Although division of labor may explain this observation, it is also possible that educators and trainers of physicians and other medical trainees, who are themselves physicians trained to preserve and save lives, do not consider the topic important enough and shy away from it.

Table 7

Departments at M. D. Anderson Hospital including Thanatology related topics as a part of their training/educational programs for populations in the hospital, 1985-86.

Populations	Comprehensive Cancer Centers					Total No.	Percent
Medical students							
Residents	PE					1	16.7
Fellows	PE					1	16.7
Staff physicians							
Nurses	PE;	C	SW	N		4	66.7
LVN's		C		N		2	33.3
Social workers			SW			1	16.7
Clergy		C				1	16.7
Patients' relatives		C	SW		PD	3	50.0
Other (specify)							
Volunteers		C				1	16.7
General Public		C				1	16.7
Church Youth		C				1	16.7
Total # (12)	3	7	3	2	1		
%	25.0	58.3	25.0	16.7	8.3		

C - Chaplaincy	PD - Pediatrics	PS - Neuropsychiatry
N - Nursing	PE - Patient Education	SW - Social Work

It is particularly surprising that thanatology education for patients' relatives is practiced in so few cancer centers. This subpopulation has, in most cases, the greatest need for such guidance and is likely to benefit most from it. Also, this healthy subpopulation may be most motivated and receptive to instruction in cancer prevention and detection practices during this crisis period.

Research: Very few cancer centers report involvement in research on reactions to death and dying. For those who do, research is limited to three subpopulations: the clergy, patients, relatives, and (in only two institutions) patients. It is surprising that no institution reported research projects about staff's reactions to, and coping with, death and dying. Research on the psychological effects of death and dying on caregivers seems uncommon. It is limited to very few institutions. Within institutions, this kind of research would involve diverse subpopulations including, among others, physicians, nurses, administrative staff, a variety of students in different educational levels, and auxiliary staff. It is striking that no research about reactions to death and dying or the psychological aspects of dying was reported with medical students,

Table 8

Departments at M. D. Anderson Hospital offering Thanatology
related lectures/symposia/grand rounds/patient education/
other activities for populations in the hospital, 1985-86.

Populations	Lectures	Symposia	Patient Education	Staffing Conference	Process Group Following Death	Bereavement Support Group	Dpt. Total	%
Medical students	PD		PE	PD	PD		2	33.3
Residents	PE; PD		PE	PD	PD		2	33.3
Fellows	PE; PD		PE C	PD	PD		3	50.0
Staff physicians	PD			PD	PD		1	16.7
Nurses	PE; PD; N	C	PE	PD	PD		4	66.7
LVN's								
Social workers	PD; SW	C		PD	PD		3	50.0
Clergy		C		PD	PD		2	33.0
Patients								
Patients' relatives						PD	1	16.7
Other (specify)								
Psychologists	PD			PD	PD		1	16.7
Child Life Workers	PD			PD	PD		1	16.7
Translators	PD			PD	PD		1	16.7
Total (13)	3; 9; 1 1	3	4; 1	10	10	1		
%	23.1; 69.2; 7.7; 7.7	23.1	30.8; 7.7	76.9	76.9	7.7		

C - Chaplaincy   PE - Patient Education   N   - Nursing
PD - Pediatrics   PS - Neuropsychiatry   SW - Social Work

residents, staff physicians, or LVN's. This survey provides no conclusions as to why this is the case. It is possible that for this kind of research to take place, an institutional framework for dealing with thanatology must first be established.

Thanatology-related activities are conducted by and for a number of departments and subpopulations at M.D. Anderson Hospital. Evidently, however, no general framework integrating these activities exists within the institution. The planning meeting for this study appears to have been the first time representatives of hospital departments found out who is involved and what is being done in this area throughout the institution. The need to create a forum for discussion of the various types of thanatology-related activities was clearly demonstrated. Creation of such a forum within a cancer center, as well as in any other hospital, would seem to be the first step in forming a unified institutional approach to the subject. An internal survey of interests, manpower, ongoing activities, and resources in and for this area would be the second step. Such a survey may also reveal quickly whether divergent philosophical approaches to the subject exist. This was clearly the case at M.D. Anderson Hospital.

A variety of thanatology-related activities take place in the department of Pediatrics at M.D. Anderson Hospital. The activities are designed to answer needs both within the department and among the populations it serves. Patients, relatives, medical staff, trainees, students, psychologists, and social workers are all intimately involved. The age of the population of patients probably accounts for both the variety of activities and the degree of involvement. It appears that thanatology-related activities are well organized and coordinated in Pediatrics. Activities in this department probably represent the best model for an institution-wide approach to the topic.

During discussions at M.D. Anderson Hospital, it quickly became evident that one group of staff members favored and emphasized providing mainly psychosocial support, employing existing supportive techniques. The other group, while not proposing any particular approach or methodology, called attention to how little objective information is available and therefore how great the need for rigorous research on the physiology of death and dying and the effects of this process on the various individuals surrounding the patient. The difficulties and resistance to carrying out such research were acknowledged. Although at times both points of view seem to present competing and often opposing philosophies, it is evident that there is need for both.

This study, the discussions surrounding its planning, and its preliminary results indicated a need to develop a forum for discussions of thanatology-related issues and activities within M.D. Anderson Hospital before an institutional approach is developed. It also clarified the need to define goals, objectives, and research methologies in thanatology both at Anderson and elsewhere.

REFERENCES

KUTSCHER, M. L., D. J. CHERICO, A.H. KUTSCHER, A. E. HANNINEN, S. JOHNSON, AND D. PEREZ. 1975. *A Comprehensive Bibliography of the Thanatology Literature.* New York: MSS Information Corporation.

SIMPSON, M. A. 1979. *Dying, Death, and Grief: A Bibliography and Source Book of Thanatology and Terminal Care.* New York: Plenum Press.

Index

Alzheimer's Disease
   in cancer patients, 187–191
   patient competency assessment, 3,
      187–191

body image, 167
   alteration of, 7
breast cancer, 125–132
   existential group therapy, 150–161
   marital interaction, 136–142
   mastectomy patients, 156–161
   psychological profile, 150–151
   social support needs, 135–136
   uncertainty, 127–131

cancer
   pain in, 39–44
cancer education, 1–2
   cancer educator, 56–59
   communication patterns, 36–38
   effects of, 8
   ethics of treatment, 34–35
   for well siblings, 92–114
   living with cancer, 5–10
   multidisciplinary approach, 5
   of children whose parents have cancer,
      60–76
   of oncology patient, 5–10
   pediatrics, 49–58
   role of tumor board, 176–181
   teachers, 162–165
   terminal phase, 10–17
   use of humor, 218–221
   videotapes, use of, 10
cancer educator
   as role model, 56–59
   teachers, 162–165
caregivers
   grief of, 206–210
   responses to dying, 207–208
   staff support, 38
   support group, 8–9, 10, 14
children with cancer, 51–55
   coping, 57
   family impact, 115–124
clinical psychologists
   oncology support group, 6–7
   role, 3–4
colon cancer, 182–186
caregivers support group, 8–9, 10, 14
   staff support, 38
caring process, 18–27
   care for versus care about, 20–21
   motivational needs, 22–23
   nursing, 19–21
   nursing behavior, 21–22

children of parents with cancer, 60–76
   educational curriculum, 64–70
   mother with breast cancer, 145–146
colon cancer, 182–186
   psychosocial care, 182–186
communication with cancer patients, 1–17
   at time of diagnosis, 2–3
   during terminal phase, 10–17
   gaps, 41–42
   holistic approaches, 2
   importance in breast cancer, 140–142
   initial contact, 2–3
   listening, 48
   on head and neck service, 162–165
   patterns, 36–38
   physicians role, 2–3
   therapeutic metaphor, 74–89
control maintenance, 46
coping
   children, 57
   mechanisms, 26–31
   with head and neck cancer, 168–170

depression, 7–8
dying process, 12–13

education. see cancer education
existential group therapy, 150–161

family and cancer patients, 115–124
   breast cancer, 142–146
   child patient, 51–56
   patient education, 5–6
   social context of breast cancer, 134–149
family
   reunion, 15
   role in terminal care, 10–11
family stress, 8–9

group process
   in pediatric cancer patient, 77–89
group therapy, 152–153
   existential, 150–161
   of terminally ill, 192–199

head and neck cancer, 166–175
   caring for patient, 166–175
   coping with, 168–170
   role of tumor board, 176–181
   service, 162–165
   tumor, 176–181
hopefulness, 26–31, 47–48
humor
   as a teaching strategy, 218–221
hypnotherapy, 6

indicators of care, 20–21
   nursing care behaviors, 20–21

intervention
    with breast cancer, 146
    rejection of, 8–9

loss therapy, 201

mastectomy patients, 125–132, 150–161
    emotional profile, 151–152
    existential group therapy, 152–153
    group therapy, 152–153

nonverbal communication, 11
nursing role, 8
    care for vs. care of, 20–21
    caring behaviors, 21–22
    caring process, 20
    staff support, 38

oncologists, 10
    pediatrics, 49–50, 53–54, 57–58
oncology family reunions, 15

pain in cancer, 39–44
    addiction, 43–44
    assessment of, 39–40
    profile of patients, 40–41
    use of narcotics, 42–44
parents
    of children with cancer, 51–55
    with cancer, 60–76
patient competency
    assessment, 3
patient education
    living with cancer, 5–10
    time of diagnosis, 2–3
patient needs, 211–217
    perceptions of family and nurse, 211–217
patient/physician relationship
    and prognosis, 28
pediatrics
    communication, 74–79
    family impact, 115–124
    mother with breast cancer, 145–146
    use of group process, 77–89
pediatric cancer education
    childrens' perceptions, 50
    educating, 56–59
    extended family, 52
    for well siblings, 90–114
    role of parents, 51–52
    teaching curriculum, 60–76
    use of therapeutic metaphor, 79–89
physician's role
    in communicating, 2–3
    pediatric cancer, 50–51

placebo effect, 29–30
psychological care, 8
psychologist, clinical, 3–4
psychopharmacology, 7–8
psychosocial care
    colon cancer, 182–186
    in pediatric cancer patients, 77–89
psychosocial
    intervention, 45–55
    needs, 8
psychotherapy, 6, 7, 12–13
    group counseling, 192–199
    group process, 77–89
    individual, 6
    loss therapy, 201
    time-limited therapy, 200–205

quality of life, 187–190

religious beliefs, 12, 29
reunions, family, 15

self-esteem, 7
sexuality, 3, 4, 10
    relation to breast cancer, 137–140
social worker
    clinical role, 4, 14–15
stress
    coping mechanism, 26–31
    self-regulatory control, 29
support groups
    caregivers, 8, 9, 14
    oncology, 6, 7, 10
    pediatric cancer patients, 77–78
    staff, 38
symptom control, 33–34

terminal care, 10–17
    dying process, 12–13
    group counseling, 192–199
    physical contact, 11–12
    religious beliefs, 12
    staff attitude, 16
thanatology in cancer centers, 222–232
    caregivers' responses to dying, 207–208
therapeutic metaphor in pediatric cancer
    patients, 78–89
time-limited therapy, 200–205
tumor boards, 176–181

uncertainty
    breast cancer, 127–131

videotapes, use of, 10